Goal-Oriented
Medical Care

Goal-Oriented Medical Care

Helping Patients Achieve
Their Personal Health Goals

James W. Mold, MD, MPH

FULL
COURT
PRESS

First Edition

Copyright © 2020 by James W. Mold

For permission requests, please address
Full Court Press
1001 Blackwood Mountain Rd
Chapel Hill, NC 27516

Published 2020 by Full Court Press
Printed in the United States of America

ISBN 978-1-946989-77-2
Library of Congress Control Number: 2020915959

Book Design by Barry Sheinkopf
(fullcourtpress.com)

Table of Contents

Appendices

Preface

"Health and happiness are the expression of the manner in which the individual responds and adapts to the challenges he meets in everyday life."

—Rene Dubos

SEVERAL COLLEAGUES AND I introduced the idea of goal-oriented care in a 1991 paper published in the journal *Family Medicine*. The idea emerged from my involvement in geriatric medicine, rehabilitation, and post-graduate medical education. It was simple and not particularly novel or innovative. Before deciding what to do, perhaps we — physicians and patients — should consider what we are hoping to accomplish. By then many fields had already adopted goal-oriented principles. Notable examples included education, business, and mental health.

Over the next 30 years, despite resistance from physicians, I became even more convinced that goal-oriented care would be an improvement over our current problem-oriented approach. Because it enables prioritization, it is better suited to both preventive care and the care of complex and aging patients. By reducing unnecessary and unwanted tests and treatments, it is likely to be more effective and less expensive. It is more positive and collaborative, and should therefore be more rewarding for both patients and physicians.

I now recognize that what seems to me to be a simple shift in mindset actually represents a major paradigm shift, and, as Thomas Kuhn pointed out in *The Structure of Scientific Revolutions*, paradigm shifts are hard to accomplish. Those within the system must first realize that a major change is necessary. For that reason, I am using this Preface to review a few of the shortfalls of our current problem-oriented approach.

The history of medicine is the story of our quest to understand how the human body works, the many things that can go wrong with it, and how to recognize and correct those abnormalities as early and effectively as possible. Modern physicians are, by nature and training, problem solvers, chosen because of our abilities in math and science. Medical school and residency prepared us to detect and fix, or failing that, to control aberrations of human biochemistry, physiology, and psychology. We believe that by doing so, we will help our patients live longer, more enjoyable and functional lives, and in most cases it works. However, as our knowledge and abilities have improved, and as the health care system has naturally evolved to support those within it, the linkage between our preferred strategies and the outcomes desired by patients has gradually loosened.

Advances in medical knowledge have now made it possible to identify and address risk factors for problems that haven't yet occurred. Risk factor reduction (i.e., prevention) has never fit comfortably within the problem-oriented model. "Health Promotion/Disease Prevention" looks odd on a problem list. Delivery of preventive services continues to be less than optimal even though physicians endorse its importance, and despite an ever-increasing number of preventive strategies, there is no accepted method for prioritizing them for an individual. As a result, patients are advised to undergo a long list of immunizations and screening tests, while more effective strategies like physical activity, nutrition education, and sleep often get short shrift.

Many of the "problems" we spend our time on — elevated blood pressure, blood glucose, and cholesterol, smoking, obesity, alcohol consumption, mood disorders, etc. — are actually risk factors, not problems. To make them look more like problems, we dichotomize them by drawing normal/abnormal lines through their distribution curves.

That tends to obscure the complex interactions of strengths and vulnerabilities that predict outcomes, which has delayed progress toward developing the computer algorithms needed to make sense of risk and resource profiles so that we can make valid individualized recommendations.

Diagnostic labeling can be harmful. Perhaps the best published example of this phenomenon was the randomized trial of blood pressure screening conducted years ago in a Canadian factory. Compared to those with hypertension in the "screened but not informed" group, those in the "the screened and advised to seek treatment" group subsequently exhibited increased absenteeism from work with no significant improvement in their blood pressures. Five years later their average salaries were lower than those in the "screened but not informed" group. In a small study conducted by my research team, individuals with recently diagnosed hypertension reported that it took them twice as long to recover from upper respiratory infections then a matched comparison group without hypertension, suggesting that they now viewed themselves as less healthy.

The interventions most often employed in problem-oriented care are those directly related to identified problems. Strategies that are not problem-specific, such as physical activity, healthy eating, mindfulness, handwashing, gun safety, and dental hygiene, are often neglected even when those strategies would be more impactful and less expensive than disease-specific strategies. The value of support, reassurance, encouragement, education, and reframing are underestimated, while the value of expert advice is overestimated.

The aging of the population has prompted efforts to define "normal aging," since without age adjustment, the length of the problem lists of older patients would be unmanageable. Even with such adjustments, many physicians resist caring for older people because of the number, chronicity, and complexity of their health problems. And organizing care around a lengthy problem list often obscures the issues of greatest importance. Viewing aging as a downhill path characterized by more and more health problems can be depressing for both patients and their doctors.

From a problem-oriented perspective, death represents the failure of medical interventions. Huge amounts of money are spent in the last weeks or months of life trying to keep people alive. Discussions of advance directives and end of life planning rarely occur until a terminal illness has been identified, and referrals for hospice care are often delayed. As a result, many terminally ill people receive more aggressive and expensive medical care than necessary or desired.

The unspoken assumption of problem-oriented care is that physical and psychological abnormalities are undesirable, so very little time is spent teaching us how to decide which problems ought to be investigated and solved. When a patient comes to us with symptoms, we try to relieve them. As a result, too many childhood ear infections are treated with antibiotics, increasing the rate of recurrence, encouraging earlier visits for subsequent episodes, and possibly contributing to the childhood obesity epidemic by altering the gut microbiome. Too many people with low back pain are addicted to narcotics, muscle relaxants, and surgical procedures. Diagnostic tests are too often ordered with little thought about whether the results will lead to improvements in length or quality of life, and older patients are unnecessarily saddled with unrealistic self-management recommendations and polypharmacy.

Physicians rarely provide enough information to their patients about how their disease-management recommendations relate to meaningful outcomes. I often wonder why patients are willing to take blood pressure medications every day for the rest of their lives without knowing how many additional months of life they are likely to gain by doing so. Perhaps that is why long-term adherence to most medications is less than 50%.

When health is operationally defined as the absence of problems, costs can be expected to increase as the health care system gets better at detecting and correcting them. In fact, that appears to be what is happening. Nearly two-thirds of recent increases in health care costs can be attributed to the increasing prevalence and detection of diseases and to new tests and treatments.

With better tests and treatments, the parameters defining "normal" will continue to tighten. Based upon the law of diminishing returns, the cost required to bring people into alignment with those narrowing parameters will increase exponentially. For example, there is no evidence that reducing the diagnostic threshold for diabetes from a fasting blood sugar of 140 mg/dl to 126 mg/dl has increased the length or quality of life of those affected, but it has almost certainly increased health care costs.

Advances in genomics and genetic reengineering threaten to bring these challenges to a head, raising questions about whether seeking normalcy is even a good idea. Are we searching for the perfect genome? If we could achieve that, would our species be able to survive? Doesn't our survival depend upon genetic diversity?

As diagnostic tests have improved, clinicians rely less and less on the information provided by patients, and standardization of treatment recommendations has reduced the perceived need to understand context. Because problems can be separated cognitively from the people who have them, a problem-oriented approach tends to dehumanize care. More insidiously, it has caused those involved in reforming the health care system to underestimate the importance of therapeutic relationships.

Just as Newtonian physics is good enough in most situations, problem-oriented care works well-enough most of the time. However, even then, understanding patients' goals and priorities and the values and preferences that underpin them almost always contributes something to patient care. In addition, the process of acquiring and using that contextual information for decision-making strengthens the physician-patient relationship, which is often vital to both short- and long-term therapeutic success.

In goal-oriented care a *goal* is a desired outcome for which it makes little or no sense to ask, "Why would you want that to happen?" *Objectives* are measurable steps along the way toward goal attainment, and *strategies* are ways to reach objectives and achieve goals. In the final year of her long life, my mother was willing to see a physical therapist and do some home exercises (strategies) in order to walk safely without a walker (objective), so that she could take care of her many outdoor plants (goal). Having a meaningful goal motivated her to work on her balance. Understanding her goal allowed me to help her explore alternative options when those efforts appeared to be failing. Our interactions around her goal brought us closer together.

Blood pressure reduction is a strategy for reducing the risk of strokes, heart failure, heart attacks, and kidney damage (objectives) in order to prevent premature death and disability (goals). Focusing on the goals could encourage a physician and patient to consider which preventive strategies would be most effective and feasible for that individual. For some patients, blood pressure reduction might be less effective than smoking cessation or physical activity. For some, blood pressure reduction might be ineffective prior to reduction of alcohol consumption.

It is important to understand that goal-oriented care is not about asking patients what they want and helping them get it. Goals, objectives, and strategies are, whenever possible, developed and agreed upon by patient and physician. Patients contribute information about needs, desires, resources, values, and preferences. Physicians contribute information about medical options, obstacles, and probabilities. Care plans are developed by considering all of this information.

Abnormalities of biochemistry, physiology, or psychology are reconceptualized as obstacles or as challenges to be faced when trying to achieve a goal. Goals are therefore established before considering whether problem-solving is a reasonable strategy. Whereas problem-solving often requires minimal knowledge of the patient as a person, goal-setting demands collaboration, a shared understanding, a mutual commitment, and a trust-based clinician-patient relationship. That requires a greater investment on the part of both physicians and patients.

A common concern among physicians is that goal-oriented care will take additional time. I hope to convince you, using clinical examples, that it probably won't. With some exceptions, the goal-directed approach actually takes less time.

Many experienced clinicians, particularly those who have cared for the same patients over many years, will discover upon reading this book that they already practice goal-oriented care but didn't know what to call it or how to explain it. On the other hand, students and residents may find goal-oriented care difficult to understand and implement because of their emersion in a problem-oriented culture. Post-training, physicians who grasp the concept may struggle to deal with system obstacles like record systems, quality indicators, and coding and billing.

I hope that the concepts presented in this book will provide a framework within which all clinicians, particularly those involved in primary care, can improve their clinical effectiveness, partnerships with patients, and enjoyment of practice. Goal-oriented care is a broad framework within which many care models and techniques can fit comfortably (e.g., patient-centered care, relationship-based care, functional medicine, and integrative medicine).

This book is divided into three sections: Principles of Goal-Directed Health Care, Obstacles and Challenges, and Practicing Goal-Directed Care.

Let's begin.

Introduction

*"The good physician treats the disease; the great physician treats
the patient who has the disease."*
—Sir William Osler, 1899

*"The practice of medicine in its broadest sense includes the whole
relationship of the physician with his patient."*
—Francis Peabody, 1927

*"[The kind of health that men desire] is the condition best suited
to reach goals that each individual formulates for himself."*
—René Dubos, 1959

FROM THE TIME OF GALEN (129-216 AD), the quests of medical
practitioners and researchers have been to discover the causes of
human suffering and death and find ways to diagnose and treat them.
Early efforts focused on figuring out how the human body worked. In
1543, Andreas Vesalius published a compendium on the subject titled
Concerning the Fabric of the Human Body. Two centuries later, Gio-
vanni Battista Morgagni published *The Seats and Causes of Diseases
as Demonstrated by Anatomy*.

As nineteenth century biologists were preoccupied with the classification of plants and animals, physician scientists were classifying diseases. The systems of the body had been characterized, and so diseases
were classified within those systems. That has continued to the present
day, the latest version, *The International Classification of Diseases –
Version 10*, having recently been released.

As medical research advanced our knowledge of both normal and
abnormal bodily structures and functions, the volume of information
became more than any physician could absorb and retain. A logical
consequence was greater and greater specialization and increasing com-

plexity of the health care system. Less obvious was the gradual shift in focus from patients to their diseases. As shown in the quotations at the beginning of this Introduction, a number of clinicians and authors noticed this trend and tried to raise the alarm. More recently, women insisted that pregnancy should not be viewed as a disease. A whole new specialty of palliative care was established to humanize end-of-life care.

In 1967, the American Academy of Pediatrics began to promote the importance of a primary care *medical home* for children with developmental disabilities and other chronic health problems. It was an attempt to emphasize the importance of having a place within the health care system where care could be coordinated over time, where clinicians were concerned about the child and not just their impairments. A pediatrician and epidemiological researcher, Barbara Starfield, established the critical importance of the generalist function, now called primary care, subsequently defined by the Institute of Medicine (IOM) as "the provision of integrated, accessible health care services by clinicians that are accountable for addressing a large majority of personal health-care needs, developing a sustained partnership with patients, and practicing within the context of family and community."

In 1969, the specialty of Family Medicine was established in an attempt to preserve generalism while embracing advances in medical knowledge by recognizing the need for additional training and a greater presence in academic medical centers. The early academic leaders of this new specialty, most of whom had been in private community practices, emphasized the importance of the human, contextual, and interactional elements of care. They adopted the biopsychosocial model of George Engel, who proposed that "interactions between biological, psychological, and social factors determine the cause, manifestation, and outcome of wellness and disease."

The first residents to enter Family Medicine residency programs were revolutionaries, students who defied the advice of their medical school faculty hoping to humanize health care. I graduated from medical school in 1974 having experienced care in both the academic medical center and several rural community settings. The contrast seemed dramatic to me, and I enthusiastically joined the revolution. Led by an eternal optimist, my residency program was filled with idealistic people trying to make the world a better place. We felt particularly good about taking care of vulnerable and underserved patients. Though we adopted the problem-oriented record system proposed by Lawrence Weed, we filed records by family. There were rocking chairs in every exam room.

Unfortunately, while the early leaders of this movement remained committed to transforming the health care system, a great deal of their energy was, of necessity, spent gaining credibility and stature within academic medical centers. Over time, compromises were made, conservatism crept in, and subsequent cohorts of faculty and trainees were more willing to accept medical care as it was taught primarily by subspecialists.

In 1984, after spending six months in West Africa followed by six years in a rural practice in North Carolina, I accepted a faculty position at an academic medical center. Nearly all of the faculty in the department had also been in private practice and had retained their desire to improve the system, but few of the residents or students were interested in challenging the standard medical model. They just wanted to get a job with reasonable hours and a good salary. It soon became clear to me that the revolutionary spirit that had attracted me to Family Medicine was waning.

However, as one revolution was petering out, another was gaining momentum. Though the field of geriatrics had existed for more than a century in Europe, it only became important in the United States in the late 1970s and early 1980s, led by the Veteran's Administration and several prominent academic programs. Our department recognized a need for geriatric teaching sites and had established a teaching nursing home service before I arrived. However, the person primarily responsible for it was leaving as I arrived.

I enjoyed taking care of older patients, and most of them seemed to appreciate my honesty and sincerity. I liked the clinical complexity as well, but mostly I was drawn to the revolutionary spirit of those involved. Once again, I found that I had joined a group of people who were trying to humanize care, and this time the revolution involved health care professionals from many different clinical disciplines as well as patients, caregivers, and patient advocates, the so-called "aging network."

I developed a geriatric inpatient rehabilitation teaching service as well as a geriatric assessment clinic, and eventually a geriatric continuity clinic all in a rehabilitation hospital setting. I obtained federal grants to establish and sustain a Geriatric Education Program, which eventually became the state's Aging Center. I completed a part-time geriatric fellowship and obtained a Certificate of Added Qualifications in Geriatrics, having passed the first certification examination in 1988.

In the rehabilitation setting I was, for the first time in my medical career, fully introduced to the idea of goals. Of course, I had been required to specify goals when making outpatient referrals for physical therapy, but I didn't really know how to do it and generally left it up to the therapists. Now I was sitting in team meetings reviewing the goals for each patient each week.

At about that same time, our department was rethinking its resident adviership process. Another physician faculty member and I met with a professional educator to design the new process. She taught us about the Individualized Education Program (IEP) used in the school system to develop educational plans for children who were struggling. Because the residency program offered a number of different training paths, individualized planning seemed appropriate. Not surprisingly, the IEP process begins with the establishment of educational goals.

I began to wonder why goal setting wasn't a core feature of medical care. I conducted a literature search and found that most of the publications came from either rehabilitation or mental health. However, there were several published studies showing that goal setting appeared to be effective in other clinical situations (e.g., diabetes management), particularly when behavior changes were required. I also found an article written by a quality improvement consultant stating that he was unable to accurately assess the quality of care provided in a hospital setting since the goals of care were so rarely stated. A faculty colleague from our School of Social Work had published a book chapter clarifying the differences between goals, objectives, and strategies.

By 1991, I had limited my practice to patients over the age of 65 in preparation for the development of a geriatric fellowship program. The more I learned from my rehabilitation colleagues, the more it seemed that a goal-oriented approach was a better way to provide care, at least for older, complex patients. I began to write an article articulating the idea. Two faculty colleagues, Greg Blake and Lorne Becker, reviewed drafts of the article and made significant contributions. The paper, which we called "Goal-Oriented Medical Care," was subsequently published in the journal *Family Medicine*. One of the observations Lorne made was that what seemed to me to be a simple idea represented a major paradigm shift.

That initial article seemed to have little impact. The editor of *Educational Gerontology* asked me to write a follow-up article on the impact of goal-oriented care on geriatrics and gerontology education. That article, titled "An alternative conceptualization of health and health care: Its implications for geriatrics and gerontology," attracted even less attention than the first one. It was referenced in a book on public health and aging, and I was invited to give a talk at Queen's College in Ontario, but that was about it. Over the next several years, I wrote several other articles and a book chapter, and I gave a number of lectures on goal-oriented care. I also began to gain experience applying it in my clinical practice.

Meanwhile, in 2005, the primary care specialty associations, for political and financial reasons, resurrected the idea of medical homes, expanding the name to *patient-centered medical homes (PCMHs)*, which were essentially primary care practices by a different name. While patients never embraced the name PCMH (it sounded too much like nursing home), it was attractive to policy-makers, payers, accrediting bodies, researchers, and frontline clinicians. A definition and criteria were developed creating a push for formal accreditation processes. Reimbursement was soon linked to PCMH accreditation, and thousands of journal articles were written about the components of a PCMH, the methods required to become a PCMH — called *practice transformation* — and the impact of PCMHs on patient and clinician satisfaction, clinical outcomes, and cost.

Once some of the practical, organizational, and financial issues had been sorted out, attention shifted to the meaning of *patient-centered*. Those efforts led to a variety of interventions. Moira Stewart, who published one of the first books on the subject (*Patient-Centered Medicine: Transforming the Clinical Method*, first published in 1995), stated in a 2001 *British Medical Journal* article that, "Patient-centeredness is becoming a widely used, but poorly understood, concept in medical practice. It may be most commonly understood for what it is not — technology-centered, doctor-centered, hospital-centered, disease-centered."

We all have ideas that seem brilliant at first blush, but less so after some time has passed. Th goal-oriented care idea was different. The more I thought about it, the better it seemed. Clinical challenges brought up in conferences, on hospital rounds, or while precepting residents were often easier to understand and address using a goal-oriented approach. It seemed to be applicable to all patients, not just those who were old or complex. Students who saw patients with me reported that there was something different and better about the way I approached patient care, though they couldn't articulate what exactly it was.

I had little difficulty teaching patients and their families to think in terms of goals, though I rarely used that word. Convincing physicians was a different matter. Students and residents were intrigued, but there were too many obstacles and few other role models. A non-physician colleague suggested I write a book for patients, hoping they would then demand goal-oriented care from their primary care physicians, but I was too busy to even think about writing a book.

I was able to convince a medical student to do a small summer research project to find out if physicians would respond to patient goals and priorities when expressed in writing on routine pre-visit forms. They didn't. That student, Becky Purkaple, became a believer, and subsequently, during her residency, repeated the study, adding a prompt for the physicians to ask patients about health-related challenges to their quality of life. The physicians again seemed unable to incorporate information provided by their patients about quality of life challenges and goals into their decision-making process. Becky is now in private practice providing goal-oriented care.

Given my growing frustration that a good idea was largely being ignored, imagine my excitement when, in 2012, an article by David Reuben and Mary Tinetti, both academic geriatricians, was published in the New England Journal of Medicine titled *Goal-Oriented Patient Care: An Alternative Health Outcomes Paradigm*. I contacted Dr. Tinetti, and we have since had an opportunity to work together to promote the concept.

In 2015, shortly after I had retired from the university, I had another wonderful surprise, a phone call from Belgium. Jan De Maeseneer, Professor and Chairman of the Department of Family Medicine and Primary Health Care at Ghent University, called to ask if it would alright if he nominated my original 1991 paper for inclusion in a book to be called *Family Medicine: The Classic Papers*. Apparently, he read the paper when it first came out and was so taken with the idea that he redesigned his residency curriculum around it. I said yes.

Also, in 2015, twenty-five years after the term was officially endorsed, Sandra Tanenbaum published an article in *Health Care Analysis* proposing a typology of patient-centered care. She was able to distinguish four types: 1) Whole patients versus their parts (i.e., holistic care; integrated care); 2) Patients versus providers (i.e., anti-paternalistic; shared decision-making); 3) Patients versus the health care system (i.e., access, convenience, care coordination; patient navigators); and 4) Patients as persons (i.e., person-centered care). The specific example she found of person-centered care was narrative medicine, a process of care that focuses on the patient's story using literary techniques to help patients make better decisions about their health and health care.

Andrew Miles and Juan Mezzich, in a 2015 article in *Health Care Analysis*, proposed that person-centered care is care "of the person (of the totality of the person's health, including its ill and positive aspects), for the person (promoting the fulfillment of the person's life project), by the person (with clinicians extending themselves as full human beings, well grounded in science and with high ethical aspirations), and with the person (working respectfully in collaboration and in an empowering manner through a partnership of patient, family, and clinician)." Jacob Eklund, in an article published in *Patient Education and Counseling* in 2019, concluded that "The goal of person-centered care is a meaningful life while the goal of patient-centered care is a functional life." Dr. Tanenbaum posited that while patient-centered care is typically viewed as a means to an end, the quadruple aim (higher quality, lower cost, better patient outcomes, and enhanced clinician well-being), person-centered care is viewed as an end in itself (humane interpersonal care).

Which brings us back to the goal-oriented care conceptual framework and my personal windmill-charging quest to make health care more humane. Over time, I discovered that the process created when patient and clinician collaborate to clarify goals and priorities, develop and attempt to carry out agreed upon strategies, is of, by, for, and with patients, an end in itself. The importance of goals lies not in their achievement but in their attributes. Goals are outcomes each person considers important and meaningful, a reflection of their values. They are aspirational rather than an effort to correct deficits. And, the goal-oriented framework comfortably accommodates scientific advances while providing a basis for prioritization.

So, if it is such a good idea, why hasn't it been universally adopted? In *The Tipping Point*, Malcolm Gladwell argues that the rate of spread of new ideas is dependent upon three major factors: a small number of key people he calls mavens, salesmen, and connectors (the law of the few), the stickiness of the idea, and the context in which the idea is proposed. Having read the book, I set about identifying key people and telling them, individually and in conference settings, about goal-oriented care. I wrote the book for patients, *Achieving Your Personal Health Goals: A Patient's Guide*, that my geriatric colleague had suggested years before and sent copies to a variety of mavens, salesmen, and connectors, though I have no way of knowing whether many of them read it.

There are some problems with stickiness. The word *goal* means different things to different people. To patients, *goal* seems too big, suggesting lofty, probably unachievable aspirations. Having figured that out early on, I avoided using the word in clinical situations. Prioritization seems to be stickier, and Mary Tinetti now calls her version of goal-oriented care, patient prioritized care. In addition, the idea can sound so simple as to seem trivial and uninteresting, simply a change in semantics. Family physicians, in particular, claim that they already use a goal-oriented approach. However, after fully grasping the concept and its implications, they often dismiss it as impossible.

For years, however, the greatest challenge has been context. By the time of our 1991 article, problem-oriented medical records had been adopted by nearly all health care providers and organizations. The electronic record systems developed since then have all used that model though most have omitted what Weed called the Personal Profile, a comprehensive narrative description of patients and their situations in life.

In 1998, Ed Wagner and his colleagues at the MacColl Center for Healthcare Innovation introduced the Chronic Care Model. The model, which was developed based upon a review of the literature and observation of exemplary practices, identifies health system and broader societal elements needed to support "productive interactions" between an informed, activated patient and a prepared, proactive practice team. The nature of productive interactions was not specified. Predictably, the mission became delivery of problem-oriented care more consistently and efficiently to populations of patients. A widely adopted innovation was disease-oriented practice registries generated automatically from the electronic record systems.

Evidence-based medicine launched in the 1980s had facilitated the development of primarily single-disease-based clinical practice guidelines (CPGs). Though the intent was to reduce unwarranted variations in practice and to protect physicians from pressure to order unnecessary tests and procedures, there were several unintended adverse consequences. Standardization taken too far led to what many doctors have called cookbook medicine, all patients with the same diagnosis treated the same, "no patient left behind."

By this time, health care had become one of the largest sectors of the U.S. economy, attracting experts in business. Rising health care costs continued to be of great concern to policy-makers and business executives. Conservative politicians became convinced that the only way to reduce health care costs was to develop new payment models and encourage competition. The result was the corporatization of health care.

A popular cost-reduction model was the health maintenance organization in which physician practices were paid a preset amount for the care of a defined group of patients with some of the money withheld in a shared risk account. However, ethical concerns were soon raised by primary care physicians particularly who were being forced to weigh their own incomes against the interests of their patients. That led in the 2010s to newer payment models like Accountable Care Organizations and Value-Based Purchasing in which value was defined as quality divided by cost. In the absence of easily monitored alternatives, quality was based upon adherence to the CPGs, further institutionalizing the problem-oriented model.

It was in this context that patient-centered care emerged as a counterforce. Patients and their advocates drove the creation of patient advisory committees in hospitals and larger practices. The Affordable Care Act established the Patient-Centered Outcomes Research Institute. Patient navigator, care coordinator, and community health worker roles have been established. Shared decision-making aids are being created. In fact, some progress has been made in all three typological areas identified by Tanenbaum. But the problem-oriented care approach has survived.

I have come to realize that Lorne Becker was right. Goal-oriented care is more than a simple idea. It represents a paradigm shift, and paradigm shifts are tremendously disruptive. They don't generally happen until all efforts to save the existing paradigm have failed. That hasn't happened yet, but it will. People are living longer. Medical advances like genetic testing and gene manipulation, engineered organs, and stem cell therapies are likely to create major financial and ethical challenges. Problem lists are destined to grow exponentially. Rationing, no matter how surreptitiously and creatively it is done, can only contain costs temporarily. More and more physicians are experiencing dissatisfaction and burnout, and patients, having had enough of assembly line care, will demand fundamental change.

This book is for the physicians who will be there when the paradigm shift occurs, and for the aging revolutionaries who never gave up hope, the younger physicians who will lead the way, and physicians of all ages who are invested in the well-being of each person in their care.

Acknowledgements

ANYONE WHO HAS WRITTEN A BOOK understands the importance of the people who provide encouragement and honest feedback throughout the process. This book would not have been written without the support and encouragement of my wife, Sandy. Partial compensation was the time I spent on my computer rather than getting in her way during the COVID-19 pandemic.

During the final two years of my Family Medicine residency program, each resident was partnered with another resident in the same year. My assigned partner was Bill Lee. We had grown up only 25 miles apart and attended medical schools 10 miles apart, but we had never met until we both chose a residency program more than 600 miles away. Though our career paths have been quite different, we have remained close friends ever since. Bill is the consummate family physician, the kind of doctor everyone hopes to find for themselves and family members. Besides being extraordinarily competent, he absolutely loves helping people. He practiced full-time for more than 40 years and still helps out in his old practice when needed. For all of those reasons, Bill was the first person I asked to review drafts of the book, and his feedback and suggestions were extraordinarily helpful.

Rick Finch was one year ahead of us in the same residency program. I was impressed by his quiet competence and willingness to teach. We have exchanged Christmas letters through the years, and he and his wife, Paula, have visited us in our home several times. Rick practiced in Washington state for more than 30 years before retiring at the age of 57. In his words, "the frustration of forcing myself into the jaws of the coding and billing machine proved more and more frustrating, and infuriating for me—a big reason for the burnout that led to my retirement." When considering who, besides Bill Lee, I wanted to receive feedback from on the book, Rick came to mind immediately. We had discussed the concept during one of his visits, and he seemed to get it right away. He agreed to be a reviewer, and his comments and suggestions have been invaluable.

When I left private practice for academic medicine in 1984, and we moved halfway across the country, one of the first people my wife and I met was Claudia Shoultz. We stayed with her and her family while house hunting, and despite a number of changes in jobs, locations, and living situations since then, we have remained close friends. Now that we live in the same state again, we are able to visit more regularly. It turns out that her husband, Donn, writes novels and short stories, nearly all of which I have read and enjoyed, and Claudia, a journalist by training, has become his editor. During a coordinated vacation on Hilton Head Island, I asked if I could pay her to edit this book. She agreed but refused to accept any money. How great it is to have good friends who are also talented!

Two and a half years ago, I was considering attending the North American Primary Care Research Group (NAPCRG) annual meeting in Chicago. Prior to retirement I had been a regular attender, but that was when I had a faculty benefits account. As I scrolled through the titles of the presentations, to my great surprise and excitement, I saw a workshop on Goal-Oriented Care. When I e-mailed the primary presenter, Agnes Grudniewicz, I discovered that she was working with another Canadian researcher, Carolyn Gray Steele, and a physician-researcher from Belgium, Pauline Boeckxstaens, to establish the research foundation for goal-oriented care beginning with a scoping review and an in-depth case study of three practice sites that had implemented goal-oriented care. I offered to help them with the workshop, and they invited me to participate. Since then, we have presented together twice more at NAPCRG and once at an exciting symposium on goal-oriented care in Belgium attended by more than 200 health and social services professionals. The discovery that so many people around the world are interested in goal-oriented care raised my level of enthusiasm for writing the book and my hope that I will live long enough to see much broader adoption of the approach. When introducing me at conferences, Agnes is fond of saying that they invited me into their group and now they can't get rid of me.

Section I

Principles of Goal-Oriented Health Care

"By health, I mean the power to live a full, adult, living, breathing life in close contact with what I love—the earth and the wonders thereof. . . . I want to be all that I am capable of becoming."
—Katherine Mansfield

"The treatment of a disease may be entirely impersonal; the care of a patient must be completely personal."
—Francis Weld Peabody

PROBLEM-ORIENTED CARE IS BASED UPON the assumption that preventing or correcting abnormalities of structure and function will allow patients to have long and rewarding lives. It is a deficit reduction approach that assumes abnormalities are undesirable and potentially correctable. The goal is normalcy.

Goal-oriented health care, on the other hand, involves helping patients define and then work to achieve their health goals. The focus is on outcomes rather than methods. Adding the goal-setting step enhances the role of the patient, strengthens the physician-patient relationship, focuses strategies on positive outcomes, and supports prioritization. Life is viewed as a journey filled with challenges and opportunities, and health is defined as the ability to successfully face those challenges and capitalize on those opportunities. From that conceptualization, it is possible to derive four types of health-relevant goals: 1) preventing premature (preventable) death and disability; 2) maintaining or improving current quality of life (ability to perform necessary functions and enjoy meaningful activities); 3) optimizing personal growth and development; and 4) experiencing a good death.

Physicians who care for individuals over many years tend to adopt a goal-oriented approach. The better we know our patients as human beings, the more we care about what happens to them. We naturally begin to focus on outcomes that are meaningful for each patient. My hope is that, by clarifying the principles of goal-oriented care, physicians can learn them from the beginning and apply them throughout their careers. In this section of the book, I will discuss each of the four categories of goals and the role of physicians in helping patients achieve them.

Chapter 1a

Prevention of Premature Death and Disability

"You have two lives. The second one begins when you realize you only have one."
—Confucius

"But what we can do is think of ourselves as something more than technicians in control of the body. At times we can be like gardeners, teachers, servants, or witnesses to the people we meet as patients."
—Abraham M. Nussbaum, M.D.

Prevention of Premature Death and Disability as a Goal

SURVIVAL IS A BASIC HUMAN INSTINCT. We all want to stay alive as long as possible unless and until we reach a point when life becomes unbearable or loses all meaning. However, most of us prefer to avoid thinking about our own mortality until it is imminent. When people consult a physician, it is most often because of symptoms that are affecting their quality of life. But quality of life is only relevant if you are alive. Therefore, one of our most important responsibilities as physicians is to make sure that prevention of premature death and disability is given appropriate weight. The reason for considering death and disability within the same goal category is that both outcomes are in the future, and, with some notable exceptions, the strategies tend to be the same (e.g., reducing the risk of a stroke reduces the risk of both premature death and disability).

When prevention of premature death and disability are viewed as goals, we are forced to consider the relative impacts of all available preventive strategies. That involves assembling for each patient a profile of risk factors, resources, and preferences, most likely causes of death, and a list of strategies prioritized based upon their probable impact on life expectancy and future disability. Given the number of risk factors and preventive strategies available to most people, these calculations can best be done using computerized algorithms, but there are some relatively simple principles that can be applied.

Biological Requirements for Human Life

When survival is a goal, one of the highest priorities is to make sure that fundamental biological needs are met. In The Finest Traditions of My Calling, Abraham Nussbaum devotes a full chapter to the idea of the physician as gardener. He wonders, "If we could reenchant medicine, perhaps we could move away from the model of physicians as technicians controlling the failing parts of a patient and allow them to be more like gardeners tending to patients."

Whether it is done for pleasure or nourishment, gardening is a goal-oriented activity, and gardeners think a lot about the basic biological needs of plants, soil, water, and sunlight. Humans also require food, water, and sunlight. In addition, we need physical activity, sleep, and a safe place to live, free from toxins and other environmental hazards.

It is difficult to assess the adequacy of a patient's nutritional intake. Some brief screening instruments have been developed (see Appendix A), and there are computer programs that calculate the nutrient content of foods consumed. Printed instructions are available online for the Mediterranean and DASH diets, which appear to be optimal for survival. Both of those diets are consistent with the conclusions of Michael Pollan in The Omnivore's Dilemma: "Eat good food, not too much, mostly vegetables." Research also supports the value of consuming plenty of olive oil, tree nuts, and oily fish like salmon, and avoiding highly processed foods and sugar. The value of intermittent fasting is still unclear.

Our daily water requirement under ordinary circumstances is the sum of urine output (around 1,500 cc for adults) and insensible loss (around 1,000 cc for adults). Almost half of that amount is obtained from food. This suggests that, absent risk factors and special circumstances, adults should try to drink at least 1,500 cc (six cups) of fluid a day (e.g. two cups with each meal or one cup with each meal and one cup between meals).

Because of the risk of skin cancers, we have been led to believe that exposure to sunlight is dangerous. In fact, *lack* of sun exposure is more dangerous. Our understanding of why sunshine is essential continues to expand. We have long understood that exposure to ultraviolet radiation contributes to the production of Vitamin D, which is important for calcium metabolism and bone formation. We now know that Vitamin D helps regulate more than 1,000 different genes impacting the function of nearly every organ in our bodies. In addition, sunlight has positive effects on immune function, production of serotonin and melatonin, neuropeptide substance P, and endorphins.

What we don't know is how much sunlight exposure is enough. Current recommendations (12 – 15 minutes per day) are based solely on requirements for Vitamin D production. Treatment of patients with seasonal affective disorder seems to require at least 30 minutes a day, preferably in the morning. Epidemiological data linking increased incidences of various cancers to greater distances from the equator suggests that more sunlight exposure may contribute to the prevention of premature death.

Aerobic physical activity is not just a way to improve cardiorespiratory fitness. It is a requirement for survival. Inactivity changes biochemical processes in ways that may have been protective in the short term (energy conservation during the winter) but are clearly harmful in the long term. Insufficient physical activity is as important as deficiencies of vitamins, minerals, or hormones. When muscles are being used, they release hundreds of signaling molecules into the bloodstream, some of which reduce intravascular inflammation, a major contributor to cardiovascular events. Other signaling molecules reduce the levels of sex hormones, decreasing the risk of some cancers of the reproductive system. Still others increase insulin sensitivity, reduce morning cortisol levels, and improve immune function.

In a 1982 article in JAMA called "Disuse and Aging," William Bortz pointed out that the changes we have come to associate with aging are remarkably similar to those caused by inactivity. For a compelling review of the biochemical changes associated with physical activity, I recommend reading *Younger Next Year* by Chris Crowley and Henry S. Lodge. Note: There are two versions of the book, one for men and one for women.

To prevent premature death, we seem to need between 90 and 150 minutes of moderately intense physical activity per week, sustained for at least 10 minutes at a time. Moderately intense physical activity is activity that raises your heart and breathing rates enough that you can still talk but not sing. In one large prospective study, adults who reported at least thirty 20-minute episodes of moderate physical activity per month (140 minutes per week) were 25% more likely to be alive 23 years later than those reporting no 20-minute episodes, after controlling for other known predictors of mortality. Since much of the life gained from engaging in physical activity will be spent engaged in that activity, patients should be advised to choose activities they enjoy. (I choose to play basketball and walking my dogs.)

Because it can affect both survival and future disability, oral health is paricularly important. Good oral hygiene reduces the risk of pneumonia, for obvious reasons, but also cardiovascular events. Gingival disease in particular increases the risk of tooth loss, hyperglycemia, preterm births, and possibly Alzheimer's Disease. Tooth loss can contribute to malnutrition and loss of confidence and self-esteem. All patients should be advised to take care of their teeth, including brushing, flossing, and regular visits to a dentist.

Gardeners have begun to recognize the importance of the many different organisms in the soil to the health of their plants and the harms that can result from over-tilling, over-fertilizing, and the use of insecticides and herbicides. Medical researchers are finding that the same principles apply to human health. Advances in DNA sequencing methods have resulted in an explosion of new information about our microbiomes. While this research is still in its infancy, we can say with certainty that our health depends upon the health of the populations of microorganisms in our mouths and guts and on our skin.

Social and Environmental Risk Factors

Just as plants do better in some settings than in others, where we live is important for survival. A person living in Summit County, Colorado (Breckenridge, Keystone, etc.) can expect to live 20 years longer on average than someone living on the Oglala Lakota Indian Reservation in South Dakota. If you live along the Mississippi River between Arkansas and Mississippi, your life expectancy is in the 60's. If you live in Southern Minnesota, it is in the 80's. Most of the differences appear to result from social, environmental, and behavioral factors, with access to health care playing a much smaller role. Lack of social support, for example, carries health risks of the same magnitude as unhealthy behaviors. In longitudinal studies, lonely and socially isolated people have a 64% greater death rate than those who are not lonely or isolated. If we are serious about longevity as a goal, educating patients about the importance of their environment should be included on our list of preventive recommendations.

Table 1a.1 lists some of the more important socioeconomic and environmental determinants of health.

Table 1a.1 Social and environmental factors that can impact survival

Income	Access to walking paths and recreational opportunities
Education	Access to public transportation
Employment	Exposure to intimate partner violence
Social support	Exposure to environmental toxins
Access to healthy foods	

Toxins

Neither plants nor humans do well when they are exposed to toxins. Children are at risk for exposure to a variety of household products that can be toxic. Older homes may contain lead in paint or in water from lead pipes. Carbon monoxide detectors can significantly reduce the risk of poisoning of both children and adults. In areas of known risk, homes should be tested for radon, since prolonged exposure increases the risk of lung cancer.

Of the various toxic substances to which people can be exposed, tobacco and alcohol are particularly dangerous because of their widespread availability and addictive potential. Cigarette smoke contains more than 6,000 different chemicals, many of which are toxic to humans, including heavy metals, carbon monoxide, nitrosamines, and polyaromatic hydrocarbons. As a result, cigarette smokers, as a group, don't live as long as non-smokers, and they often die of uncomfortable conditions like cancer and chronic obstructive lung disease. Epidemiological data suggests that each cigarette smoked reduces a person's average life expectancy by 11 minutes. For a one pack per day smoker, that is a loss of nearly two months of life per year of smoking. A one-pack-per-day smoker has an average life expectancy at least ten years lower than a nonsmoker.

Alcohol is also a broad-spectrum toxin. There is some debate about whether the harms outweigh possible cardiovascular benefits from small amounts of alcohol (2 drinks per day for men and 1 drink per day for women). The latest epidemiological data suggests that there is no safe amount and that each drink above one per day reduces life expectancy by an average of about 15 minutes. A man who drinks three standard-sized drinks (See Table 1a.2) per day therefore loses an average of nearly eight days of life per year, and the adverse effects per drink aregreater for women. In moderate drinkers, the excess deaths appear to result from strokes and heart failure. Heavy drinking increases the risk of various cancers, hepatic cirrhosis, and pancreatitis as well as accidents, homicides, and suicides.

Table 1a.2 Alcoholic beverage amounts considered to be one standard-sized drink

Beverage	Amount
Beer with 5% alcohol	12 oz (one regular-sized can/bottle)
Beer with 7% alcohol	8.5 oz (3/4 of a regular-sized can/bottle)
Beer with 9% alcohol	6.7 oz (1/2 of a regular-sized can/bottle)
Wine with 12% alcohol	5 oz (5/8 cup; typical serving of wine)
Wine with 15% alcohol	3.8 oz (<1/2 cup)
Wine with 17% alcohol	3.6 oz (<1/2 cup)
Distilled spirits with 40% alcohol (80 proof)	1.5 oz (1 shot glass)

When taken as directed, opiates are less toxic than cigarettes and alcohol, but when misused, they can be lethal. Unintentional overdoses in particular have become a huge problem in the U.S. Cocaine is another cardiotoxin that is commonly abused. Methamphetamine is also a systemic poison with high addictive potential. We now have effective tools for identifying and helping patients with tobacco, alcohol, and illicit drug usage.

Greater attention is now being paid to a wide variety of less obvious chemical toxins. Information on environmental toxins is reported regularly by the CDC—(see https://www.cdc.gov/exposurereport/index. html.) However, recommendations for what physicians should do to educate, screen, and advise patients is still limited. Expect that to change in the coming decade.

Finally, prolonged sitting has recently been shown to be toxic to human beings separate and apart from deficiency of physical activity. In post-menopausal women, for example, every hour of sitting per day is associated with a 7% increase in insulin resistance, a reflection of systemic intravascular inflammation.

Addiction

Addiction is the result of a biochemical alteration in the brain, which can be extremely difficult, though not impossible, to correct. When it occurs, it has a negative impact on all four health goals and should therefore be a top priority for physicians and patients.

The relative addictive propensities of nicotine, heroin, cocaine, alcohol, caffeine, and marijuana are shown in Figure 1a.1.

Figure 1a.1. Addictive propensities of commonly abused substances

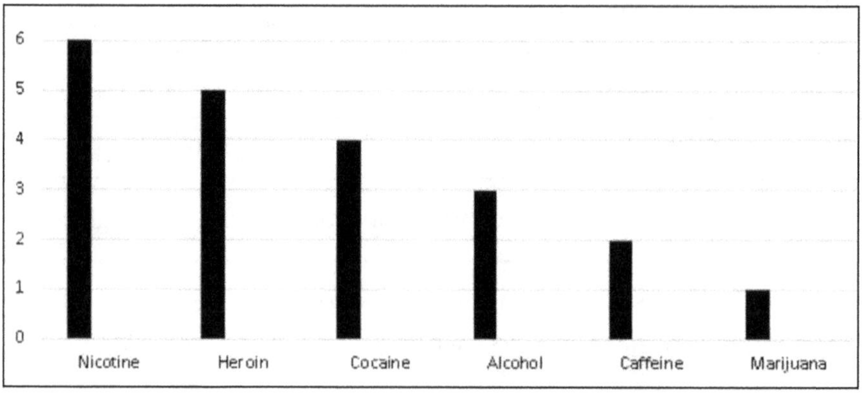

Humans can become addicted to virtually anything that causes pleasure, particularly when the pleasure follows soon after the behavior or event and dissipates just as quickly. Behavioral addictions can be just as harmful and hard to reverse as addictions to cigarettes, alcohol, and drugs. Examples include addictions to eating, gambling, money, the internet, video gaming, shopping, sex, risky behaviors, plastic surgery, achievement, and work.

Trauma

Both physical and psychological trauma are other preventable causes of death. Accidents and injuries are the fourth or fifth leading cause of death in the U.S. Guns kill more children and adults than motor vehicle accidents. Individuals living in homes with guns are three times more likely to die of suicide and more than twice as likely to die of homicide than those living in gun-free homes. Seatbelts, motorcycle and bike helmets, smoke detectors, fire extinguishers and safe storage of firearms are simple, effective risk reduction measures. Multiple, repetitive adverse childhood experiences can reduce life expectancy by as much as 20 years.

Patient Education

You may be thinking, "Don't most people already know these things? Do I really need to spend my limited time on things that ought to be handled by public health or the school system?" If the goal is to prevent premature death, the answer is yes.

Several years ago, my research team received a contract to develop an interactive telephonic program to help patients concerned that they might have the flu. As part of the evaluation, we asked for user feedback. One person wrote, "The information provided was very helpful. For example, I didn't know that handwashing could prevent the spread of my infection."

Sometimes a message is simply more effective when it comes from a physician. Even though nearly everyone now knows that smoking is harmful, physician advice to quit remains one of the most effective smoking cessation strategies.

Although many patients seem to want to believe that they have complete control of the choices they make in their lives, we know that each of us has vulnerabilities and propensities based upon our genetic makeup, epigenetic traits, and life experiences. When we all have our DNA mapped and analyzed, genetic vulnerabilities will be easier to identify. Until then, it is our responsibility to obtain an accurate family history when possible and counsel patients about potential susceptibilities and how to mitigate them. In my garden I use leaf mulch around my plants to inhibit weed growth and diatomaceous earth to hinder insects because I know my plants are susceptible to those threats.

Common Causes of Death

Based upon death certificates, the most common causes of death in the United States are those listed in Table 1a.3.

Table 1a.3. Ten most frequent causes of death based upon death certificates

Cause of Death	Number of Deaths in 2016	Percentage of All Deaths
Heart Disease	633,842	24.1%
Cancer	595,930	22.7%
Chronic Lung Disease	155,041	5.9%
Accidents and Injuries	146,571	5.6%
Alzheimer's Disease	110, 561	3.9%
Diabetes mellitus	79.535	3.0%
Influenza and pneumonia	57,062	2.2%
Kidney Disease	49.959	1.9%
Suicide	44.193	1.7%

However, we know from autopsy studies that the proportions of deaths caused by heart disease, respiratory disease, and diabetes are probably somewhat lower and the numbers of deaths from trauma, suicide, and gastrointestinal problems are likely higher than reported. In addition, according to the 1999 National Academy of Medicine report, *To Err is Human*, medical errors account for between 44,000 and 96,000 deaths. Since most iatrogenic deaths occur in the hospital, patients should do everything possible to avoid hospitalization and, when hospitalized, they should ask a family member or other caregiver to be there to guard against errors.

Behavioral Risk Factors

More important than those final causes of death are the risk factors underlying them. Unhealthy behaviors, including use of tobacco products and alcohol, unhealthy eating, and lack of physical activity together contribute to up to 50% of premature deaths. Smoking alone contributes to 20% of all deaths in the United States. Physicians know this, of course, but we often put too little time and effort into helping patients adopt healthier behaviors for several reasons. Most of us weren't trained to provide effective behavioral counseling, and it is somewhat less rewarding than other clinical activities because it takes time and the results may not be seen for months or years. We also don't have a quantitative measure of the impact of our efforts, and insurance companies tend to pay us comparatively less for counseling visits.

Most importantly, we have failed to collaborate with researchers and public and mental health professionals to develop effective community-based systems to support healthy behaviors. But, if one of the most important goals is to prevent premature death and disability, helping patients choose healthier behaviors should be one of our top priorities.

While prevention of premature death and disability is the most important reason to address unhealthy behaviors, in my clinical experience, an essential first step to behavior change is to help patients identify a compelling quality of life goal.

Several years ago, my colleagues and I interviewed a number of people who had been able to lose at least 10% of their body weight and keep it off for more than a year. In every case, those individuals mentioned a quality of life goal as the primary motivation. They told us that:

1. The first thing they had to do was "get their head on straight," meaning they had to make a conscious decision that they were going to change their eating and activity habits for the rest of their lives.

2. They made that decision in order to be able to do something they viewed as important (e.g., live to see their grandchildren grow up, run marathons) or avoid something they found intolerable (e.g., not be an embarrassment to their family, not have to take medications for diabetes and high blood pressure). In other words, they tied their behavior change to a quality of life goal. For the most part, their quality of life goals were compelling and relatively long term, something important enough to carry them past temptations to return to prior behavior patterns for the foreseeable future.

3. They found a method that they could believe in and that they felt they could stick to for the long haul. This often took a period of trial and error.

4. They enlisted the help of family members or significant others to encourage them during hard times.

5. They forgave themselves for short-term lapses, and they rewarded themselves when they were able to sustain their healthy behaviors through difficult periods.

6. Finally, they reported that their primary care physicians helped them by providing information, encouragement, and advocacy.

The problem-oriented medical approach to overeating includes labeling it—we now have specific categories: overweight, obese, and morbidly obese — and prescribing dietary modifications, physical activity, and sometimes medications or surgery. The goal-oriented approach begins with a discussion of goals, followed by an assessment of resources (family support, access to healthy foods, ability to exercise, etc.), then thoughtful consideration of possible strategies, and then, if all requisite conditions are met, a trial. The chosen quality of life goal is front and center throughout the process and at every follow-up visit.

Even when all of the necessary requirements are met, it may take multiple attempts over several years to help people change an unhealthy behavior. Sometimes all you can do is plant a seed and hope it takes root.

Screening

Screening for preclinical conditions, while less effective than primary preventive strategies, is still valuable for many patients. It is important to remember that screening recommendations are based upon average benefits and harms across the population, and that while the size of the benefit (i.e., numbers of lives saved) may be substantial from a public health perspective, it may be trivial for an individual.

In addition to the criteria that must be met before a screening test is sanctioned by the United States Preventive Services Task Force (USPSTF), the following conditions should also be met before recommending a screening test for a patient: 1) the probability that the patient has the condition must be great enough to outweigh the risks associated with that test; 2) they must be willing to pursue further testing or treatment if the test is positive; 3) the benefits of further testing and treatment would likely outweigh the potential harms; and 4) their remaining life expectancy must be long enough for the benefits of screening to be realized.

Table 1a.4 summarizes how long it takes, on average, to benefit from some common screening tests.

Table 1a.4. Years required to benefit from common screening tests

Purpose of Screening	Time Required for Benefit to Exceed Harm
Cervical Cancer	5–7 years
Breast Cancer	10 years
Colorectal Cancer	10 years
Prostate Cancer	10–15 years

However, using this information to help patients make good decisions can be tricky. I had a patient who was 90 years old and was accustomed to having a colonoscopy every ten years. He was reluctant to accept that his life expectancy had decreased to the point that he would probably not benefit and would more likely be harmed by the procedure. After all, he had lived longer than his previous physicians had predicted, outliving many of them.

Another patient of mine was 75 years old when he had an elevated screening prostate specific antigen test ordered by another physician. He was referred to a urologist who was reluctant to proceed with biopsies because of his age. The urologist asked me to estimate the patient's life expectancy, which, based upon his overall medical condition and risk factors, I estimated to be about 8 years. Apparently, the urologist then told the patient that he didn't need further work-up because I had said he wouldn't live long enough to benefit. The patient fired me. He said he didn't want a doctor who expected him to die in 8 years.

Addressing Chronic Health Challenges
Appropriate management of chronic health challenges can reduce the risk of premature death or disability from a little bit to a great deal.

Chemotherapy for certain types of advanced cancer can extend life by several months; treatment of patients with systemic lupus erythematosus with hydroxychloroquine can extend life by several years; and dialysis can often increase life expectancy by a decade. When developing a prevention plan, it is important to try to clarify the size of the impacts of available strategies as well as their potential adverse effects on quality of life so that patients can make informed decisions about what they are willing to do to achieve the expected benefits.

Prioritization

The potential impact of a preventive strategy depends upon each patient's unique set of risk factors. Consider the case of Mr. Sawyer, a 68-year-old retired welder. A widower, he lives in an apartment by himself. He requires supplemental oxygen 24 hours a day because of emphysema. Despite that, Mr. Sawyer still enjoys his somewhat limited life, which includes reading, television, e-mailing friends, and going out to eat three times a week at a cafeteria close to his apartment. His two children and four grandchildren visit him nearly every week. He quit smoking several years ago, has had influenza and pneumonia vaccinations, and is correctly using the inhalers that his doctor recommended for emphysema based upon the results of his pulmonary function tests. He has an electric stovetop and a housekeeping service and is not exposed to excessive fumes, dust, mold, or mildew.

Based upon current guidelines for the medical management of stable emphysema, Mr. Sawyer is following all appropriate recommendations. Additional guideline recommendations include physical activity as tolerated and consideration of nutritional supplements if there is evidence of malnutrition. Consideration should be given to whether he might benefit from lung volume reduction surgery or a lung transplant.

It would also be helpful to know which of the available treatment strategies prolong life and which are palliative. For example, is there any evidence that inhaled bronchodilators have a positive or negative effect on longevity or are they only for symptoms, in which case, perhaps he should try stopping them periodically to see if they are still required.

What else could Mr. Sawyer do to prolong his life?

Focusing on the goal -- prevention of premature death -- rather than the strategy -- management of chronic lung disease -- provides a different view, revealing additional strategies. The logical first question to ask is, "From what is Mr. Sawyer likely to die?" The answer, I suspect you will agree, is pulmonary failure precipitated by infection. That being the case, how could we help Mr. Sawyer avoid respiratory tract infections?

Strategies for preventing infections include reducing exposure to infectious agents and strengthening resistance to their initiation and impact. To reduce exposure to viral pathogens, Mr. Sawyer should tell family members not to visit when they are symptomatic and commit to washing his hands after touching surfaces others may have touched (e.g., in the cafeteria). He could reduce his exposure to bacterial agents by practicing good oral hygiene and having his teeth cleaned by a dental hygienist every six months. Since H2 blockers and PPIs appear to increase the number of bacteria in the trachea and the risk of bacterial pneumonia in patients with chronic lung disease, he should avoid those if possible.

Resistance to respiratory infections requires a good cough reflex, adequate pulmonary secretions and ciliary activity, and immune responsiveness. This suggests that Mr. Sawyer should understand the importance of good hydration and nutrition. Multivitamin/mineral supplementation could be considered. ACE inhibitors tend to increase the cough reflex and have been shown to reduce pneumonia rates in at least one clinical trial involving stroke patients, so that could be considered, particularly if inadequate coughing is a concern.

Mr. Sawyer's case is somewhat unique in that his most likely cause of death is clear. However, the most probable cause of death for each of us could theoretically be calculated from population statistics and our unique risk factor profile. While inaccuracies in cause-of-death statistics and incomplete information on the impacts of risk factors and preventive strategies limit the accuracy of such calculations, it is possible to identify major threats, particularly as patients age and begin to develop chronic health challenges. A goal-oriented approach will encourage researchers to gather better data and develop more accurate and helpful ways to analyze it.

The concept of prioritization should be familiar to most physicians. It is the approach used by financial advisors. It is likely that, at some point, your advisor asked you a series of questions having to do with your assets, liabilities, values, preferences, and goals, plugged the answers into a computer, and produced a set of recommendations. I am still upset that my financial advisor forgot to ask me to consider the cost of two out-of-state university educations and my daughter's wedding. We could take the same approach to prevention of premature death and disability, but it would require the same kind of computer program. Now consider the case of Frances Warren.

Mrs. Warren is a 55-year-old black married woman with a college education, a full-time job and an average household income. She lives in an urban area. Her body mass index is 25.4, and her diet includes lots of salt, red meat, and fried foods. She smokes one pack of cigarettes per day and engages in no regular significant physical activity. She drinks alcohol only occasionally. Her average blood pressure is 160/90, and she has mildly elevated total (260 mg/dl) and LDL (160 mg/dl) cholesterol levels and a borderline low HDL cholesterol level (45 mg/dl). Both parents have elevated blood pressure, and several relatives have experienced strokes. She has had a Pap smear within the last three years, a mammogram in the last two years, and a flu shot this year.

Based upon her risk factors, she can expect to live to be 66.4 years of age, and she can expect to spend the last 2.5 years of her life disabled. In Table 1a.5, I have listed a variety of preventive strategies available to her and the estimated impact of each of them on her life expectancy.

Note: The estimates were generated by a computer program developed by Zsolt Nagykaldi at the University of Oklahoma that uses a proportional hazards equation developed from population statistics, adjusted for more than 200 possible risk factors and the impact of recommended preventive strategies on each of them.

Table 1a.5. Selected preventive services recommended for Francis Warren and their impacts on her life expectancy

Preventive Strategy	Estimated Years of Life Gained
Smoking Cessation	6.5
Moderate Physical Activity	3.8
Blood Pressure Reduction (130/80)	2.2
Statin	1.1
Healthier Diet	1.1
Colorectal Cancer Screening	<0.5
Lung Cancer Screening	<0.1
Total (Doing All of the Above)	**15.2**

If one of her goals is to avoid premature death and disability, Mrs. Warren and her physician should put a great deal of effort into smoking cessation and increasing physical activity. In fact, because of the law of diminishing returns (See Chapter 1b), if she were to stop smoking and engage in recommended amounts of physical activity, the total additional benefit of blood pressure reduction and a statin would be reduced to 1.1 years.

Why not do everything on the list? There are at least two reasons. Kimberly Yarnell and her colleagues calculated that providing all of the primary and secondary preventive services indicated for every patient seen in a typical primary care practice would take 7.4 hours per working day, and providing guideline-recommended care for patients with chronic illnesses would add another 10.6 hours. Similar time and energy limitations apply to patients. In addition, greater benefits accrue from focusing on the most impactful strategies, especially if those strategies are difficult or time and energy intensive. Once the most impactful strategies have been accomplished, the others can then be considered.

Doing Only What is Necessary

In addition to focusing attention on probable causes of premature death and disability and ways to prevent them, a goal-oriented approach highlights strategies that are unlikely to be helpful.

A personal friend, Dora Menninger, celebrated her 101st birthday this past year. She was living in her own home, completely independent at that time. She began to have trouble getting out of bed, unable to make her legs work properly. She was able to call her daughter, who took her to the local hospital emergency room.

For several years Dora had been treated for lumbar spinal stenosis. Since no other cause was found, spinal cord and nerve root compression due to spinal stenosis was believed to be the most likely cause of her acute problem. However, since she needed additional imaging studies and a neurosurgical evaluation, and because she was now unable to care for herself, she was admitted to the hospital.

On admissionl, Dora's blood pressure was 180/90, so she was given medicine to lower it. That medicine lowered her blood pressure enough to reduce the amount of blood reaching a vulnerable area of her brain.

The result was a stroke that left Dora paralyzed on one side of her body and unable to speak. After months of physical, occupational, and speech therapy, she moved into an assisted living center where she lived for two more years, substantially disabled.

The only reason to lower blood pressure is to prevent premature death and disability. In the absence of heart failure or an aneurysm, blood pressure reduction is a long-term risk reduction strategy. In the Systolic Hypertension in the Elderly Program (SHEP) study, blood pressure reduction over a period of 4.5 years resulted in 5.5% fewer cardiovascular events and 1% fewer deaths. The benefit of reducing Dora's blood pressure for a few days while in the hospital, or for the remainder of her life (estimated life expectancy of two years), was negligible, too small to warrant taking any risk at all.

Acute Life-Threatening Conditions

Every physician needs to be prepared to recognize and treat or refer patients with acute life-threatening conditions. Undergraduate and graduate medical curricula should include as a priority information about, training in, and experience with treatable life-threatening conditions, both common and rare. Most of these conditions fall within the categories of infections, traumatic injuries, bleeding and clotting disorders, mental health conditions, a few serious metabolic disorders, and toxins.

Prevention of Future Disability

Factors that increase the risk of premature death are generally the same ones that cause disability. Therefore, most preventive strategies apply to both. However, some of the most common causes of disability don't necessarily result in premature death. The most common causes of long-term disability in the United States are musculoskeletal disorders, including arthritis, back pain, and injuries; cardiovascular problems; and mental health and other neurological disorders, including sensory loss.

Chronic low back pain causes more total years of disability than any other single condition. In the 2009-2010 National Health and Nutrition Survey, chronic low back pain was found to be associated with less than a high school education, low household income, and obesity. Other risk factors include exposure to occupational hazards (e.g. heavy lifting, bending, twisting) and a family history of back problems. Unfortunately, there is little information on how to prevent future disability due to back pain. However, it seems reasonable to alert patients to the risk and to educate those at high risk in proper lifting techniques and avoidance of particularly hazardous activities if possible. Spinal cord injuries are uncommon but more disabling. The most common causes are motor vehicle accidents, falls, acts of violence, and sports and recreational injuries.

Nearly all meaningful activities require a functioning brain. Therefore, strategies that enhance and preserve brain function are especially important. Formal education, reading, socialization, and lifelong learning improve brain function in both the short- and long-term. A number of activities are associated with a substantial risk of brain injury. Those risks can be reduced somewhat with protective headgear, but short-term enjoyment should also be weighed against the risk of future disability.

Impairments of vision, hearing, taste, smell, and proprioception can also reduce quality of life. Regular eye examinations, use of noise reduction devices, and avoidance of physical and chemical injuries to the tongue and nasal passages seem reasonable. Patients are most likely to agree with such recommendations when they are tied to the activities they value.

From Compliance to Adherence to Collaboration

When medical care was largely paternalistic, patients were expected to follow the advice of their doctors. If they didn't, they were considered to be noncompliant. As care has become more collaborative, the word, noncompliance, has morphed into non-adherence, a slightly softer term. Neither is germane to goal-oriented care.

In goal-oriented care, agreement on goals and strategies is a collaborative process. Neither doctor nor patient has all of the relevant information. Decisions are complex, and initial plans are rarely perfect. Finding the best path to better health generally involves a series of adjustments made based upon lessons learned over time. Take, for example, the case of Thomas Washington.

When I met Mr. Washington, he had been admitted to the hospital three times already that year for congestive heart failure due to systolic dysfunction. The residents on the inpatient team had correctly determined that the reason for the hospitalizations was that Mr. Washington did not always take his heart medicines. However, they had been unable to figure out why. One of them even speculated that he enjoyed being in the hospital.

I found Mr. Washington to be a very pleasant, if reserved, man with at least average intelligence. He had no trouble engaging with me or answering my questions. Our conversation went something like this:

Me: I understand that you've had this same trouble before with fluid buildup. The other doctors who've seen you think it's because you don't always take your heart medicines.

Mr. Washington: Yes, sir. I suspect that's right.

Me: Can you help me understand why that happens?

Mr. Washington: OK. What can I tell you?

Me: Why don't you start by telling me where you live and what a typical day is like for you?

Mr. Washington: Well, I live on the eighth floor of a high-rise apartment building about five blocks from here. I generally get up and take a shower, then get dressed and have a little breakfast. There's a senior citizen center on the first floor. I generally go down and spend the morning there playing dominoes or checkers. You know. They serve lunch and have some kind of program. Then I go up to my apartment, take a nap, watch TV or read the paper, fix my supper, watch some TV, and go to bed.

Me: So why don't you always take your heart medicines?

Mr. Washington: Well, see there's not but one bathroom at the senior center and lots of people in line to use it. When I take the heart medicine, I have to pee a lot, and when I have to go, it can't wait, so sometimes I decide not to take it.

Me: So why don't you take the medicine in the afternoon, after you get back to your apartment?

Mr. Washington: The doctors told me I had to take it first thing in the morning.

Me: That was just so you wouldn't have to get up in the night to pee.

Mr. Washington: Getting up at night wouldn't be no problem for me.

Me: Then you could start taking all of your heart medicines when you get back up to your apartment after visiting the senior center. Do you think that would work better for you?

Mr. Washington: Yes, sir. It surely would.

The initial plan had been reasonable, but it had not been adjusted once Mr. Washington identified having difficulty with it.

Trade-Offs

It is rarely possible to reduce the risk of premature death without risking a reduction in quality of life. Moving to a safer neighborhood cuts ties to significant people and places. Reducing blood pressure with medication often involves additional expense, inconvenience, side effects, drug-drug and drug-nutrient interactions, and adverse labeling effects. Acknowledging the trade-offs allows patients to make informed choices.

Several years ago, my primary care physician advised me to begin taking a statin to lower my LDL cholesterol. At the time I wasn't taking any medicines and considered myself to be extraordinarily healthy. I also had (probably) irrational fears that statins might reduce my muscle strength and my ability to continue to play basketball based upon one small study I had read. Before I was willing to decide, I needed to calculate and then weigh the approximately 3% reduction in 10-year risk of a cardiovascular event against the cost, inconvenience, and known and unknown side effects of statins.

Final Thoughts

Good gardeners know that all the insecticides and fungicides in the world won't prolong the life of a plant living in poor soil with too little water and sunlight. It is time for physicians to focus on what matters. A goal-oriented approach in which prevention of premature death and disability is a priority will encourage physicians and their patients to do that more strategically and effectively.

Viewing prevention through a goal-oriented lens tends to broaden the range of potential strategies and helps physicians and their patients individualize and prioritize them. Reframing diseases as risk factors consolidates primary, secondary, and tertiary preventive strategies, which makes it easier for patients to understand the purpose and benefits of our recommendations. Social and environmental determinants of health and disease are simply additional risk factors. Genomics will continue to add to the list, and computer-assisted risk assessment will become even more essential.

Good gardeners know that plants need lots of tending. Unpredictable changes in weather, weeds, and predators require adjustments to best-laid plans. In patient care, adjustments in care plans are equally important, expected, and essential to goal achievement. In fact, the reassessments and adjustments are often more important than the original plans of care.

Chapter 1b

The Law of Diminishing Returns

"The law of diminishing returns means that even the most beneficial principle will become harmful if carried far enough."
—Thomas Sowell

How Much Risk Reduction is Enough?

THE *LAW OF DIMINISHING RETURNS,* first described by economists, explains why, under certain circumstances, additional inputs produce smaller and smaller outputs. Applied to risk reduction, the law of diminishing returns posits that once high impact strategies have been implemented, subsequent strategies will result in smaller and smaller benefits for the patient.

There is a simple mathematical explanation. Absolute risk reduction (ARR) is the product of preintervention risk (R) and the relative risk reduction (RRR) produced by an intervention [ARR = (R) (RRR) (100%)]. If, for example, a patient's 10-year heart attack risk is 20% and high-dose statin therapy can reduce that risk by 30%, then the ARR will be 0.2 X 0.3 X 100% or about 6%. If a second, equally effective risk reduction strategy is then initiated, its proportional impact is applied to the new preintervention risk of 14%, resulting in an ARR of only 4.2% (0.14 X 0.3 X 100%). Each successive strategy has a smaller and smaller impact as the preintervention risk is reduced.

We now have many ways to reduce the risk of major adverse cardiovascular events (MACE), events that often result in death or disability. Some interventions reduce risk more than others. It can be shown mathematically that, if the most impactful ones are implemented first (e.g. smoking cessation, physical activity, blood pressure reduction, and statin therapy), the first three or four strategies will generally lower MACE risk enough that additional strategies will have a negligible impact. That is good news. It means that patients don't have to do everything to obtain near maximum benefit.

The law of diminishing returns also applies to risk factors that are continuous rather than dichotomous. For example, in patients with systolic blood pressures (SBP) of 200, lowering their SBP from 200 mmHg to 180 mmHg will have a larger effect on risk of stroke than lowering it from 160 mmHg to 140 mmHg, and while there is still some benefit from lowering it further, from 140 mmHg to 120 mmHg, it is very small. Remember though that reducing the risk of heart attacks and strokes is an objective, not a goal. The goal is to reduce the risk of premature death and disability. Depending upon an individual's overall risk profile, lowering systolic blood pressure may have a larger or smaller effect.

Rational prioritization is complicated. Determining optimal combinations of strategies will require sophisticated computer programs and better data on causes of premature death and disability. However, the implications of the law of diminishing returns can still improve the effectiveness of our recommendations while reducing unnecessary interventions.

Why Not Do Everything?

An oft forgotten component of the law of diminishing returns is reflected in the last part of the quotation at the beginning of this chapter: "… will become harmful if carried far enough." It isn't just that the benefits of successive interventions are reduced. There is also danger that recommending too many interventions can be counterproductive or even dangerous.

One of my frustrations with physical therapists is that they tend to recommend so many different exercises that patients find they are unable to do them all, and so they give up and do none of them. My approach, in those cases, was to ask patients how many they thought they could do regularly, and then help them choose what appeared to be the most important ones within those limits.

The same principle can be applied to medications. The more different medications prescribed for a patient, the greater the chance they will take them incorrectly or not at all. In addition, increasing the number of medications increases the number of potential adverse effects and interactions. While there is considerable individual variability, the rates of incorrect use and adverse effects and interactions tend to increase exponentially once the total number of different medications exceeds five.

Prioritization

It almost always makes sense to implement the most effective preventive measures first. Once that has been accomplished, other measures often become more important. Said differently, once the probabilities of the most likely causes of death have been reduced, other causes of death become more likely, and the applicable risk reduction strategies become more important. For example, the following are computer-generated estimates for a 50-year-old white married woman with the following significant risk factors:

- Sedentary lifestyle
- 1 pack-per-day cigarette smoker
- 4 alcohol-containing drinks per day
- BMI 30
- BP 160/90
- LD cholesterol 165
- Hemoglobin A1c 8.5

Table 1b.1. Computer-generated estimates before and after implementing the most effective preventive strategies

Before	
Est. years of life gained by implementing all preventive strategies	11.91 years
Est. years of life gained by implementing each preventive strategy	
Smoking cessation	6.0 years
Moderate physical activity	3.5 years
Reduce alcohol intake to 1 drink /day	1.7 years
Reduce BMI to 24	0.6 year
All other preventive strategies	0.11 year
After	
Est. years of life gained by implementing all remaining preventive strategies	3.51 years
Est. years of life gained by implementing each preventive strategy	
Statin	1.4 years
Flu shot annually	1.2 years
Blood sugar control	0.6 year
Increase sleep time	0.2 year
Blood pressure reduction	0.1 year
All other preventive strategies	0.01 year

Notice that nearly all of the benefit initially can be obtained from the combination of four strategies: smoking cessation, physical activity, reducing alcohol consumption, and losing weight. However, once those strategies have been implemented, the patient's life expectancy is increased by almost 12 years, their risk of dying early from cancer has been reduced, and they are more likely to die of a heart attack, stroke, or influenza. At that point, a statin, blood pressure reduction, and annual flu shot become more important.

Risk Assessment

The law of diminishing returns applies to risk assessment as well. When calculating a patient's risk of dying from a heart attack, for example, many risk factors can be considered, and more are added each year. Each factor adds precision to the risk estimate. However, when chosen well, each additional risk factor adds less and less additional precision, which raises the question of how precise the estimate needs to be. The answer depends upon how close the estimate is to the intervention threshold, the level of risk that would change risk reduction decisions. As a practical matter, simple risk calculations, using combinations of no more than six risk factors, are usually good enough.

Multicomponent risk prediction tools are most useful for conditions that have multiple contributing factors. The best risk prediction tools generally include one or more measures of each of the factors contributing to the adverse outcome. Table 1b.2 lists some of the factors that can contribute to heart attacks and three commonly used risk prediction tools.

Inclusion of additional risk factors to these risk prediction tools has not been found to add significantly to their predictive accuracy or value.

Diagnostic Certainty

The law also applies to diagnostic testing. In his article, "Diminishing Returns on the Road to Diagnostic Certainty" published in 1991 in the Journal of the American Medical Association, Horton A. Johnson used diagnostic testing for iron deficiency anemia in children

Table 1b.2. Factors contributing to heart attacks and their use in risk prediction tools

Risk Factor Categories	Framing-ham	ACC/AHA ASCVD	Rey-nolds
Presence of Coronary Artery Disease			
Age	*	*	*
Gender	*	*	*
Diabetes Mellitus		*	*
Family History			*
Coronary Artery Calcium			
Carotid Artery Intima Media Thickness			
Ankle Brachial Index			
Causes of Coronary Artery Damage			
Damage Hypertension	*	*	*
Smoking	*	*	*
Homocysteine			
Causes of Abnormal Coronary Artery Repair			
Inactivity			
Lipids	*	*	*
Lipoprotein (a)			
Causes/Measures of Coronary Plaque Fragility			
Obesity			
Lipids	*	*	*
High Sensitivity CRP			*

and myocardial infarction in adults to illustrate how little information is gained by adding additional diagnostic tests once the probability of disease reaches levels above 80 to 90%.

Of course, the level of diagnostic certainty required depends upon the intervention threshold, which is the level of certainty required to initiate therapy. However, within a goal-oriented framework, there is an additional layer of complexity. Since the focus is on patient-relevant goals, it is important to first decide whether an abnormality is relevant; that is, whether a diagnosis is required in order to achieve the goal.

When my father was hospitalized for cardiac ischemia and congestive heart failure, his stool test was positive for occult blood. His blood counts were fine, and he was taking low-dose aspirin at the time, which had caused his stool tests to be positive before. His physician suggested a colonoscopy, which, on my advice, he refused. With a left ventricular ejection fraction of 30% after having had two bypass operations and a mitral valve tightening procedure, I told him that the probability that he would die from colon cancer or a remediable bleeding polyp or vascular abnormality was smaller than the probability of his dying from the colonoscopy.

Diagnostic Labeling

Diagnostic labeling ("giving someone a diagnosis") can help clinicians make assumptions about causation, treatment approaches, and prognosis. However, it can also be harmful to some patients. Within a goal-oriented framework, labeling is viewed as a strategy to be applied only when it is likely to contribute to goal achievement. The value of a patient's problem list diminishes as the number of problems on the list increases. As a geriatrician, I found long problem lists to be depressing for me, my patients, and the residents I was training. Long problem lists, in fact, are a major reason physicians are loathe to become geriatricians.

Final Thoughts

An understanding of and appreciation for the law of diminishing returns is essential to goal-oriented care. When properly applied, it can reduce the number of unnecessary interventions, make those chosen more effective, and reduce adverse effects and health care costs.

Chapter 2a

Improving Health-Related Quality of Life

"The quality of life is determined by its activities."
—Aristotle

"The pharmaceutical industry is redefining and relabeling as medical problems calling for drug intervention, a wide range of human behaviors which, in the past, have been viewed as falling within the bounds of normal trials and tribulations of human existence."
—Henry L. Lennard

QUALITY OF LIFE IS THE ISSUE of greatest concern to most people on a day-to-day basis. Though affected by many factors, health clearly plays a major role. Through a problem-oriented lens, health-related quality of life (HRQoL) is assumed to be fine (non-negative) until threatened by health problems. From a goal-oriented perspective, HRQoL is a positive construct determined by the ability to participate in essential and meaningful activities. Essential activities are activities required to comfortably get through each day, while meaningful activities are chosen activities that give life value, meaning, and purpose.

Essential Activities

Essential activities include activities of daily living (e.g., bathing, dressing, toileting/continence, eating, transferring, and mobility) and at least some instrumental activities of daily living (e.g., preparing meals, shopping, managing money, managing medications, using the telephone, and doing housework), depending upon the setting and level of support available. The most useful way I have found for identifying problems with essential activities is to ask patients to walk me through their typical day.

Mrs. Palmer was an 80-year-old widowed, retired schoolteacher who was living alone in her own home. I became her primary care physician when her prior physician moved out of state. He was evaluating her for weight loss and some abnormal liver tests, both of which had stabilized with no identified causes.

When I asked her to tell me about a typical day in her life, she said, "I get up quite early, around 6AM, go into the bathroom, wash myself off with a washcloth (it's easier than taking a shower), and then get dressed. That takes a while because it takes me about 45 minutes putting on my socks and shoes." I stopped her at that point and asked why on earth it took so long for her to put on her socks and shoes. She said that arthritis in her hips and knees made it hard to bend far enough forward to reach her feet. "It doesn't hurt. I just can't bend my joints."

Because of my experience working in a rehabilitation setting, I knew to refer Mrs. Palmer to an occupational therapist, who, in one 45-minute session, taught her how to use a sock donner and a long-handled shoehorn. With those two pieces of adaptive equipment, she was able to finish dressing in less than ten minutes. That led, at her next visit, to a discussion of bathroom equipment to make it easier for her to take a bath or shower.

The problem-oriented approach to Mrs. Palmer's arthritis would probably have unfolded in one of the following ways. Since she was not complaining of pain, it might not have been addressed at all, or it might have simply been listed on the problem list in her medical record based upon physical findings. If she had mentioned stiffness or trouble walking, her doctor might have ordered some X-rays and lab tests, which would have confirmed the diagnosis of osteoarthritis. Management might then have included acetaminophen or an anti-inflammatory medication, injections, and eventually referral to an orthopedic surgeon, measures which would probably not have improved her daily life as much as the occupational therapy referral.

Tragically, Mrs. Palmer was talked into knee replacement surgery several years later by a well-meaning family member who was concerned about her awkward gait. Postoperatively she developed a complete compartment syndrome and ended up having an above-knee amputation. She subsequently defied the expectation of her orthopedist by learning to use a prosthesis. A year later, when she developed pneumonia with an antibiotic-resistant organism, I was surprised to learn that she had listed me as her surrogate decision-maker.

Meaningful Activities

Meaningful activities are sometimes called advanced activities of daily living (AADLs). They vary greatly among individuals and are best identified with questions like, "What do you do for fun?" or "What activities are most important to you, without which life would be less meaningful?" or "What would you like to be able to do that you can't do now?" or "What does a really good day look like for you?"

Jeremy was a 33-year-old engineer who, at the insistence of his wife, made an appointment with her primary care physician, a close colleague of mine, to discuss a shoulder problem he'd had for more than a decade. The problem began with a high school sports injury. He had been a baseball pitcher, but his sports career had been cut short because of the injury to his shoulder. Since high school, he had continued to experience intermittent pain, which had prompted him to see various health professionals over the years, including several primary care doctors, an orthopedic surgeon, and a physical therapist. Jeremy had tried a corticosteroid injection, periods of rest, heat, and ice, a variety of exercises, and anti-inflammatory medications, each of which helped, but only temporarily. The orthopedist had offered to perform surgery, but he also said he couldn't guarantee that the shoulder would be significantly better afterward. After reading about the length and nature of the recovery period following rotator cuff surgery, Jeremy decided not to have the operation, at least not for a while.

Jeremy's new primary care doctor took a different approach. He began by asking, "How does the pain affect your life? What does it keep you from doing?" Jeremy reported that the most important thing he was unable to do as a result of the shoulder problem was to hunt deer with a bow and arrow, a hobby he had acquired as a teenager and had shared with his father and brother prior to the shoulder problem. "It really hurts to pull back on the bowstring." Then, it was as if an imaginary light bulb switched on in Jeremy's mind. "You know, I've seen some hunters using crossbows," he said. "I could probably do that, but I think I would need a doctor's note saying that I'm unable to use a traditional bow." His doctor wrote the note, and soon Jeremy was enjoying bow hunting again.

Once essential and meaningful activities have been identified, it is often helpful to ask why those activities are important to the patient. Understanding the values underlying goals and priorities can often open up additional strategic options, such as alternative activities compatible with the same values. A patient who wanted badly to have a dog for companionship and because of his concern about mistreatment of animals. He was unable to own a dog because his landlord wouldn't allow it. However, he was able to volunteer at the local Association for the Prevention of Cruelty to Animals chapter.

Maximization vs. Deficit Reduction

Problem-oriented care encourages patients to aspire to be normal, with no identifiable health problems: a deficit reduction approach. By contrast, goal-oriented care encourages patients to maximize their participation in and enjoyment of life.

There is no theoretical limit to the amount of pleasure or meaning a person can derive from life, and it is almost always possible to improve performance. At least that is what I tell myself every time I play basketball. While helping people find activities that provide pleasure and meaning may be beyond the scope of our job as health care professionals, we are often able to help people improve their ability to derive pleasure and meaning from the activities they choose.

Cory was a 36-year-old insurance salesman in a small town who, during a routine medical examination, asked whether there was a medicine he could take to improve his memory. His job required that he remember the names of his clients so that he could greet them by name when he ran into them in stores and other public places. It seemed to him that many of his work colleagues were better at this than he was. His mini-mental status examination score was a perfect 30. After his physician explained how aerobic physical activity stimulates brain cell growth and development, Cory joined the local YMCA and began an exercise regimen. He also bought and read a book on how to remember names and began to practice the recommended techniques. At his next wellness exam, he reported that his memory had indeed improved.

Examples of medical specialties that employ a goal-oriented approach include Sports Medicine and Physical Medicine and Rehabilitation (PM&R). Two concepts from PM&R have been particularly relevant to me: the distinction between impairments, disabilities, and handicaps, and the SPREAD mnemonic.

Rehabilitation Principles

Impairments are biological abnormalities that may impact physical functions. Hemiparesis, loss of a limb, and spinal stenosis are examples of impairments. An impairment, if significant, can result in a *disability*, the inability to perform an essential or meaningful activity. A disability, however, does not have to result in a *handicap*. People with hemiplegia can learn to cook one-handed, amputees can use prosthetics, and individuals with spinal stenosis can learn to live in a wheelchair if necessary. Whether or not a disability results in a handicap often depends upon the ability of the individual to learn new skills, use adaptive equipment, and modify their environment.

Rehabilitation therapists (e.g., occupational therapists, physical therapists, speech therapists, orthotists) are experts in helping people with disabilities avoid becoming handicapped. Of the rehabilitation therapists, occupational therapists are most accustomed to using a goal-oriented approach. However, even they can sometimes slip inappropriately into problem-solving mode.

While I was attending on the geriatric inpatient service in our rehabilitation hospital, I happened to wander into the Activities of Daily Living Room when one of my patients was engaged in his occupational therapy session. He had experienced a stroke that had left him with a right hemiparesis. He was standing at a stovetop moving modified pots and utensils around with his left hand. I remarked, "I didn't know you liked to cook," to which he replied, "I don't." "Then why are they teaching you to cook one-handed?" "I guess I failed the cooking test," he said with a hemiparetic smile.

While physicians are most comfortable treating diseases and their symptoms, the SPREAD mnemonic reminds us that helping patients improve their quality of life often requires that we not only provide SPecific treatment for the underlying condition, but also Prevent secondary complications, employ REhabilitative principles, and help patients Adapt to any remaining disabilities so they don't become handicaps.

Specific treatment implies both curative and symptomatic treatment. Prevention typically involves ensuring that the basic requirements for life and health are met (nutrition, hydration, physical activity, sleep, connection, autonomy, competence, etc.) and exposure to toxic substances and injuries are avoided during the recovery process. The range of rehabilitative strategies continues to expand, and the evidence supporting them is becoming stronger. Adaptation can include alternative ways to perform an activity, the use of adaptive equipment, and modification of the environment in which an activity is performed.

Symptoms: Acute and Chronic

Most acute symptoms are an appropriate response to a physical challenge. Nasal drainage, cough, diarrhea, and urinary frequency, for instance, help us rid our bodies of infectious agents, toxins, and other irritants. Pain and swelling help stabilize extremities following an injury and provide a healing environment. While none of us wants to be uncomfortable or have our routines disrupted, most acute, self-limited illnesses have very little impact on the four health goals, and there is often nothing much we can do about them anyway.

In the absence of preexisting health issues, acute upper respiratory tract infections including rhinitis, pharyngitis, laryngitis, sinusitis, otitis media, pharyngitis, and bronchitis almost always resolve without specific treatment in a week or two. They only shorten a person's life if complications develop such as pneumonia or meningitis, and those unusual complications almost never develop during the first five to seven days of illness. Whether the predominant pathogen is a virus or a bacterium, antibiotic treatment has little effect on recovery time, and giving our bodies a little time to respond can reduce the risk of future infections. Over-the-counter remedies are designed to interfere with normal physiologic responses. Visits with patients early in the course of such infections should therefore focus on issues other than whether the cause is a virus or bacterium and which medications will help.

Jane was an 18-year-old college student who came to see her primary care physician because of an acute upper respiratory tract infection. She had been coughing, sneezing, and feeling generally rotten for four days. Her cough was initially non-productive, but now she was coughing up small amounts of light yellow phlegm. Several of her friends had had the same symptoms earlier. Prior to this illness Jane had been asymptomatic and able to participate in her classes and intramural sports. She did not smoke or drink excessive amounts of alcohol. She had taken acetaminophen and an over-the-counter cold medicine without benefit. She wanted to get better before her next round of exams and in time to play in an intramural basketball tournament.

On the assumption that equipping Jane to handle this and future similar infections was the goal, Jane's physician expressed empathy and provided reassurance, then checked to see if she needed a note documenting her illness for school. He explained the importance of cough as a way for her body to get rid of the infectious agent. He then initiated a conversation about factors that might have predisposed her to infection like lack of sleep, poor dietary habits, and stress. They also discussed the ways that respiratory infections spread and the importance of handwashing. They agreed upon a recovery plan that included rest, fluids, no medicines, and a follow-up phone call or appointment if her symptoms were not improving in another three days.

Of course, symptoms also alert us to health challenges requiring investigation. Chronic, persistent symptoms can alert us to deficiencies of nutrients, physical activity, sleep, personal relationships, or the toxic effects of a medication, tobacco, alcohol, or psychological stress. They can also alert us to other significant health challenges. Viewed through a goal-oriented lens, symptoms are considered within the context of the goal(s) they could impact. The first priority, assuming survival is still a goal, is to determine whether the symptoms are due to a life-threatening condition. If not, the issue of concern is whether and how they are affecting or might affect important activities and what, if any, actions are indicated to either improve quality of life and/or enhance growth and development. A useful question is, "How is your symptom affecting your ability to do the things you want to do?"

Remember Mr. Washington, the man with congestive heart failure whose medication schedule needed to be adjusted so he could attend senior center activities? When I asked him what else he would like to be able to do, he said that he would love to be able to walk two blocks to the drugstore to visit the pharmacist and a couple of friends. He was prevented from doing so by shortness of breath and a tight feeling in his chest when walking that distance. No benches were available along the desired walkway. I devised a strategy involving sublingual isosorbide dinitrate, taken right before walking, and I arranged for him to obtain a cane with a built-in seat. With those two interventions he was able to get to and from the pharmacy several times each week. We also discussed additional cardiovascular event risk reduction options.

Pain

A large proportion of clinician-patient encounters involve concerns about pain. Every medical student memorizes the list of diagnostic questions a clinician should ask – onset, location, radiation, character, severity, constancy, relieving/exacerbating factors, accompanying symptoms — to determine the cause. The problem-oriented pathway then proceeds from differential diagnosis, to further evaluation and testing, to a specific diagnosis, to consideration of treatment options, and to a treatment plan. Unstated assumptions are that pain is abnormal and should be relieved whenever possible, and that pain relief will result in a return to normal functioning and improved quality of life. There is no compelling need to understand what the patient needs or wants to be able to do.

Additional questions addressed during a goal-oriented evaluation include: 1) How is the pain affecting your ability to perform essential and meaningful activities? 2) How has your life changed since you have had the pain? 3) When we reduce the amount of pain you are having, how will your life be different? 4) What do you hope to be able to do once you have less pain? Questions relevant to the patient's future life course would include: 1) Is the discomfort likely to reoccur, and, if so, what can be done to prevent it? and 2) Does the patient know what to do if it happens again?

John was a 45-year-old married man who lived on a homestead he had created in an effort to become completely self-sufficient and leave a minimal environmental footprint. However, he suffered from chronic, intermittent low back pain, which made it difficult to manage his garden and animals. He acknowledged that he was anxious and sometimes depressed, but he was adamant about not taking medications unless absolutely necessary. Aside from his age, there were no red flags suggesting that his pain was caused by an infection or cancer. I found no evidence of a structural or localized abnormality on physical examination. A complete blood count, urinalysis, and sedimentation rate were normal.

As he valued reading and continuing to learn, I suggested that he purchase Robin McKenzie's book, Treat Your Own Back, and that he try doing the recommended exercises for three weeks. I also referred him to a psychiatric social worker for cognitive behavioral therapy. At his return appointment, he was much improved. Both the exercises and the therapy had helped. Three months later, he said he had a better understanding of how the back pain could serve as a sign that he needed to employ the stress reduction techniques he had learned.

When chronic pain is viewed as a problem, the solutions are directed at pain relief. Medical visits tend to focus on medication dosing and pain contracts. Focusing on quality of life goals has two obvious benefits. Setting functional goals can provide motivation to work harder on the strategies required for improvement. At the same time, pursuing goals encourages patients to focus their attention on something other than their pain. Discussing goals can change negative conversations about refills and dosing into more positive, forward-looking ones.

What Kinds of Help Are Most Helpful?

Symptoms are typically composed of physical triggers amplified by personal fears and cultural expectations. They can trigger positive behavior changes or initiate a negative feedback loop (e.g., pain leads to reduced activities followed by dysphoria and increased pain, etc.). Symptoms can be used to avoid personal growth or as a way to exert power in relationships. How we think and feel about our symptoms can determine their impact on our lives and the lives of those around us. For those reasons, it is often as important to determine the meaning of the symptoms to patients and their families as it is to determine their cause.

Martha was a 48-year-old woman who came to see me because of diffuse musculoskeletal pain and fatigue. The rest of her medical history and examination were unremarkable. When given an opportunity to talk about her quality of life, she told me about her son, now 26 and still living at home. His failure to launch had created friction between her and her husband. He wanted to kick their son out, and she was afraid he wouldn't be able to make it on his own. I listened, expressed empathy, and attempted to reframe her situation in terms of her son's developmental needs. I ordered a few laboratory tests and asked her to return in a week. The tests were all normal, and at her return appointment her symptoms had largely resolved. She had been able to have a good conversation with her husband, and plans were underway to help their son become independent.

Experienced physicians know that the most effective interventions for non-life-threatening health challenges are often supportive listening, empathic responses, encouragement, reframing, and education. Though these approaches have rarely been compared to other therapies in clinical trials, when they have, the results have been noteworthy. For example, encouragement (e.g., "You're doing really well! Everything looks good so far!") was compared to sublingual nitroglycerine in patients with coronary artery disease undergoing graded exercise testing.

Encouragement was associated with increases in both subjective (time to development of angina) and objective (time to development of EKG changes) results equal to or greater than those seen with sublingual nitroglycerine.

Medications to Improve HRQoL

Nearly all over-the-counter and most prescription medicines available today are designed to provide symptom relief. People are encouraged, even expected, to seek treatment, usually medications, for the symptoms they are experiencing. The biggest beneficiaries are the pharmaceutical companies; the benefits to patients are often meager at best.

Pharmaceutical companies know that most people are, by nature, goal-oriented, and they use goal-oriented messages to promote their products. Ads show before-and-after sequences where people who had been sitting are now walking their dogs after taking the company's arthritis medicine, or they show a person with multiple sclerosis engaged in a variety of physical activities, as a narrator says, "Imagine what you could do with fewer recurrences."

However, these companies also exploit the fact that we have been taught to think of our bodies as broken machines, even to the point of inventing new diagnoses with catchy acronyms to convince us that we need to consume their products. Recent examples include premenstrual dysphoric disorder (PMDD), overactive bladder syndrome (OBS or OAB), hypoactive sexual desire disorder (HSDD), menopausal sexual dysfunction (MSD), and opiate induced constipation (OIC).

What they are banking on is that by giving common symptoms a diagnostic label, the symptoms will be viewed as more significant, more treatment worthy. In an ad for an expensive medicine used to treat dry eyes, the actress/patient says that she was content to live with the symptoms until she learned that she had a disease (dry eyes syndrome).

Experts have estimated that three times as many children are given the diagnosis of attention deficit hyperactivity disorder than actually have the condition, and most of them are being treated for years with potentially hazardous amphetamine derivatives. Much of the fault for this lies with the pharmaceutical industry, which has capitalized on the fears of parents that their children are at risk of falling behind their peers unless they take their medicines.

The typical pharmaceutical sales pitch includes three messages: (1) your symptoms are caused by a disease with a name (and an acronym), and 2) you shouldn't have to tolerate the symptoms because 3) there is a disease-specific treatment available — just ask your doctor to prescribe this powerful new medicine. This practice has been called "disease mongering," a term introduced by Lynn Payer in her book, *Disease-Mongers: How Doctors, Drug Companies, and Insurers Are Making You Feel Sick*. Ray Moynihan calls it "selling sickness" in *Selling Sickness: How the World's Biggest Pharmaceutical Companies are Turning Us All into Patients*.

When long-term medications are warranted to address symptoms that are interfering with HRQoL, patients should understand that you are prescribing them for that purpose and not because they will help you live longer. Knowing that a prescribed medication might improve their ability to engage in key activities increases commitment to the plan. Armed with this information, patients also know what to expect if they decide to stop taking the medicine at some point in the future. When medicines are used to both improve HRQoL and prevent premature death or disability, relative impacts on each goal should be discussed.

The Placebo Effect

In most clinical trials involving medications, about two-thirds of the positive effects are also seen in the control group. We have come to recognize this phenomenon as the placebo effect, and we tend to dismiss it as interesting but not particularly useful clinically.

Research suggests that the placebo effect appears to work through three related mechanisms, 1) belief and expectation; 2) social learning; and 3) reinforcement and conditioning. Wayne Jonas, former Director of the National Institutes of Health Center for the Study of Complementary and Alternative Medicine and author of *How Healing Works*, has suggested renaming this the "meaning response." He and other thought leaders have come to view the meaning response not as a temporary delusion, but as a physiologic process, which we all can use to recover from illnesses and injuries, one that skillful physicians can also employ to help their patients overcome health challenges.

The brain influences virtually all bodily functions, including repair and regeneration of injured tissues. When a person feels confident in a particular treatment, and that confidence is reinforced by the experience of others and by improvements in symptoms, changes occur in the brain that have a positive effect on systemic repair processes resulting in both the perception of improvement and actual improvements in bodily functions. The process need not involve medications.

The practical implications are that interventions will be more effective when patients:

- Understand the connection between a treatment and their personal goals;
- Believe the intervention is feasible and will work; and
- Have a support network that will reinforce their belief in the treatment.

In addition, according to Dr. Jonas, interventions are likely to be more effective when repeated frequently (e.g., three or four times a day), consistent with the principle of operant conditioning.

Prioritization

A major advantage of goal-oriented care is that it provides a rational basis for prioritization. That is particularly helpful in situations when the health challenges a patient faces are multiple, chronic, or complex.

"Gig" Peterson was a 65-year-old married man who, when first seen by me, was taking 12 different prescription medicines for hypertension, diabetes mellitus, congestive heart failure, chronic renal insufficiency, and gout. He was being seen by a nephrologist, an endocrinologist, and a cardiologist as well as emergency department physicians for frequent acute problems. He had recently discontinued several of his medications because of a diffuse rash.

When I asked about his usual activities, he reported that he was able to take care of himself pretty well, but he was having trouble baiting his fishing hook and taking fish off of his lines because of painful tophi. Frequent urination caused by his diuretics was also a problem for him when fishing, and he wanted to know why he had to take so many different medicines. He wanted me to help sort through them and tell him what he absolutely had to take.

His examination revealed a mildly elevated blood pressure (145/92), acute and chronic bilateral lower extremity edema with weeping venous stasis dermatitis below his knees, and gouty tophi primarily involving his fingers. Recent lab tests included an elevated BUN with near normal creatinine, an elevated uric acid, and an A1c of 7.8%

After reviewing the sequence of events leading to his current treatment regimen, several things became clear: 1) his rash was probably caused by allopurinol; 2) diuretics had had little effect on his lower extremity edema; and 3) he was taking a non-steroidal anti-inflammatory agent (NSAID), which was almost certainly contributing to his renal impairment and edema. We agreed to focus on his ability to do what he truly loved, fish, and on two objectives: 1. reduce the pain and tenderness in his hands caused by the gouty tophi and 2. reduce the number of medicines he was taking, especially the medicines that were contributing to his urinary frequency.

Over the next month, we were able to reduce his medications from 12 to 6. Discontinuation of his NSAID and reduction in his diuretic dose resulted in less urinary frequency, better renal function, less edema, and some reduction of his serum uric acid level. Topical treatment with corticosteroid cream and periodic elevation improved his venous stasis dermatitis. He agreed to try febuxostat to further reduce his serum uric acid level in hopes that his tophi would shrink. I also referred him to a hand surgeon to see if the tophi could be surgically removed if necessary, but he tolerated the febuxostat, and his tophi became less painful.

Focusing on Mr. Peterson's priorities helped us agree on a plan that he was able to understand and follow. It felt like we were on the same page.

Overdiagnosis

The purpose and most appropriate use of diagnostic labels is to facilitate communication among health care professionals. Because labeling has been shown to have detrimental effects, it should not be used when communicating with patients unless the benefit clearly outweighs the risks. The diagnosis of innocent heart murmurs in babies, even when effectively explained, results in parental overprotectiveness. The diagnosis of attention deficit disorder has benefits for some and adverse effects on others. Likewise, it isn't always necessary or wise to even pursue a precise diagnosis.

A number of years ago, while giving a talk at a national conference, my voice completely gave out. I couldn't make a sound for 15 or 20 minutes. When I got back home, I saw my primary care physician, who referred me to an otorhinolaryngologist. After a laryngoscopy, he said my vocal cords looked fine, and he sent me to a speech therapist. Based upon my symptoms, she suggested a more sophisticated test, which involved videotaping the movement of my vocal cords.

Since I wasn't thrilled about having my vocal cords examined again, I asked her what she thought might be wrong. I can't remember the name of the rare disorder she mentioned, but I do remember asking how that condition was treated. She said that if it was the problem she was concerned about, nothing much could be done, to which I replied,

"Then I'd rather not know." Her response was, "But we need a diagnosis." I respectfully (hopefully) disagreed, refused the procedure, and suggested to her that we assume it wasn't that condition. She reluctantly agreed, and my voice returned to normal with better treatment for my allergies, stress reduction techniques, and sips of water before and while lecturing.

For more information on the subject of overdiagnosis, I recommend the excellent book by H. Gilbert Welch called *Overdiagnosed: Making People Sick in the Pursuit of Health*.

Palliative Care

Because the health care system was doing an inadequate job of caring for patients with terminal illnesses, the field of palliative care emerged and eventually separated, to some degree, professionally and financially, from other forms of care. In goal-oriented care, maximizing HRQoL is an important goal of everyone throughout life. When prevention of premature death is no longer a goal, preserving HRQoL becomes predominant. That makes certain strategies more acceptable, such as the use of potentially addictive medications. Acceptance of death is an important developmental milestone and planning for a good death assumes greater importance when it is imminent. But it isn't necessary to wait for a terminal illness to begin working on those things. Goal-oriented care would obviate the need for a separate field of palliative medicine.

Trade-Offs

Just as life-prolonging measures can reduce quality of life, strategies to improve quality of life can reduce life expectancy. For example, medicines that make patients feel better can also affect their alertness or reaction speed (e.g., antihistamines, pain medications, and muscle relaxants), increasing the risk of death from a car accident or fall. Antibiotics used to treat a self-limited infection like bronchitis or sinusitis can encourage the growth of antibiotic-resistant germs, which could cause a serious and difficult-to-treat infection in the future. A goal-oriented approach doesn't resolve these conflicts, but it can help to clarify the trade-offs.

Mr. Menninger was an 88-year-old retired minister who had developed Alzheimer's disease. He also had high blood pressure, high cholesterol, aortic valvular stenosis, and atrial fibrillation. He was referred to me by his cardiologist, who had provided excellent problem-oriented medical care. When I met Mr. Menninger, his cholesterol level was normal. His heart rate was well-controlled, and he was on all of the right anticoagulant and blood pressure medications, but his quality of life was terrible, and it was getting worse. In addition to memory loss, he was lightheaded to the point of falling, and he was too drowsy to sit in church without falling asleep. His wife was afraid to take him for a walk for fear he would fall and she wouldn't be able to get him up. He was no longer able to make even simple decisions.

Mrs. Menninger was certain that her husband would not want his life to be extended, particularly since his dementia was going to continue to progress. We therefore focused our efforts on improving his quality of life. Stopping his blood pressure medicines reduced his lightheadedness and improved his ability to stay awake. There were no more falls. He rejoined his Sunday school class and was even able to give the closing prayer. He lived another year in relative peace and happiness before dying of complications of his heart disease. There is, of course, no way to know for sure whether he would have lived longer had he continued to take the blood pressure medicines, but the trade-off seemed worth it.

Stuff Happens

Despite our efforts to keep things the same, circumstances inevitably change. At some point most of us will have to give up activities we once enjoyed. When that happens, we spend some time grieving. Fortunately, life provides so many options, we can almost always find other meaningful activities to take the place of the ones we have lost.

Having said that, it is often possible to continue most activities despite advancing age or disabilities. Sometimes it is simply a matter of being persistent and finding others with similar limitations. When I retired and moved back to North Carolina, I hoped to continue to play basketball. I had heard about basketball leagues for seniors. However, when I searched the internet, I found no relevant information. I joined the YMCA and played with 20 to 30-year-olds for more than a year, struggling to keep up and frustrated that I wasn't getting the ball.

I met a few others who expressed the same frustrations, and, through them, I learned that one of the key local figures in senior basketball lived right next door to me. (Apparently old people don't advertise on the internet). He directed me to a number of men my age who were playing regularly. I now play twice a week with people who don't palm the ball when they dribble or travel when driving for a layup, remember what a set shot is, and, best of all, pass the ball.

The Importance of Understanding QOL Goal(s)

Clarification of quality of life goals often opens up an array of strategies much wider than those related to problem-solving. Sometimes activities can be modified (e.g., pickleball rather than tennis) or adaptive equipment can be employed (e.g., wheelchair basketball). Sometimes identified health problems are simply irrelevant.

Adam Ziegler was an 80-year-old retired attorney who had seen an orthopedic surgeon for neurogenic claudication due to lumbar spinal stenosis. His impression of the surgeon's conclusion was that his condition would gradually get worse, and there was nothing that could be done to treat it. When I first saw him, he was convinced that he was terminally ill. My first question to him was, "How important to you is being able to walk?" He said, "Not that important. To be happy, I need to be able to read, write, and use my computer." I then asked,

"What if you had to get around in a wheelchair?" He said, "That wouldn't be a big problem." "Then," I said, "there is no reason to be concerned about your spinal problem. The worst that could reasonably happen, and it might not, is that you would have to use a wheelchair to get around." He began to cry, and then he thanked me over and over again. Two years later, when he died of a lymphoma, he left more than $600,000 in his will for geriatric research.

Knowing that Mr. Ziegler wanted to be able to read, write, and work on his computer not only made it possible for me to reassure him about his back, it opened the door to a wide range of potential strategic options, both current and preventive. For example, it might have been helpful for him to learn about optimal seating, lighting, and eyewear options. It would have been particularly important to advise him about ways to preserve his vision. Viewing reduction of back pain as our goal would have significantly limited the range of strategic possibilities.

Chapter 2b

The Threshold Principle

"We are too much accustomed to attribute to a single cause that which is the product of several, and the majority of our controversies come from that."

—Justus von Liebig

"It is the last straw that overloads the camel."

—Asian proverb

HEALTH CHALLENGES RARELY HAVE a single cause. We are all subject to thousands of vulnerabilities and risk factors. We are born with some, and we acquire others over the course of our lives. When enough predisposing factors are present, or when individual factors are significant enough, a threshold is exceeded, and our health is challenged. This is called the threshold principle. Most physicians are familiar with the concept of a seizure threshold. The same principle can be applied to nearly all health challenges.

People who experience migraines know that a variety of factors can precipitate a headache, including stress, foods, medicines, change in barometric pressure, lack of sleep, bright lights, odors, hunger, and hormonal changes. However, they may not be aware that most of their headaches are the result of combinations of these factors, and that any single factor, by itself, is not usually strong enough to cause a headache. In fact, given the combination of enough risk factors of sufficient strength, most of us would have a migraine. People who suffer frequent migraines either have more, or stronger, contributing factors, or they have a lower headache threshold.

Even conditions that are the result of single genetic mutations can be thought of in this way. During my clinical career I took care of many people with sickle cell disease. All of these patients had the same genetic mutation, but some died in childhood, others were hospitalized repeatedly, others avoided hospitalizations but were disabled, but others grew up, completed their education, got married, and held regular jobs. How can these different outcomes be explained? The answer is that while all of these patients had the same major predisposing factor, the genetic mutation, other factors like income, education, family and social support, and coexisting health challenges had an impact as well.

The best way I have found to apply the threshold principle clinically is to make a list of all of the factors that could be contributing to a patient's health challenge, and then identify the factors that can be reduced or eliminated. While it is not often possible to address all of the factors on the list, addressing some of them — even if they aren't the most significant ones — can reduce their combined impact, hopefully below the threshold for the challenge we seek to address.

Some years ago, I took care of an 80-year-old widow who was experiencing frequent falls. She lived alone in her own home, which she and her late husband had purchased 50 years earlier. Her goal was to continue to live independently in that house, even if it meant taking certain risks. Together, she and I made a list of all the factors that might be contributing to her falls — medications, arthritis, environmental hazards, poor vision, calloused feet, worn-out shoes, etc.

Then I helped her address the factors that we could address, including a referral for cataract surgery. The eye specialist called to say that, based upon the density of her cataracts, the surgery could be delayed a while longer. When I explained that the cataracts might be contributing to her falls, he agreed to remove them. After adjusting her medications, removing environmental hazards, getting better shoes, and having the surgery, she was able to remain in her home until her death from other causes. She never, to my knowledge, suffered another serious fall.

When achieving a quality of life goal requires reducing the frequency of a symptom or event, application of the threshold principle can be quite helpful. Combinations of strategies with different mechanisms of action are often the best way to reduce a bothersome symptom. For example, in a patient with thoracic radicular pain exacerbated by muscle tension, the combination of meditation, yoga, heat, and gabapentin might help even if none of the individual measures have made any difference when used alone.

The principle can also be applied to the treatment of life-threatening illnesses. In order to develop bacterial pneumonia, a sufficient quantity of pathogenic bacteria, usually from around the teeth, must be aspirated into one or both lungs, fail to be cleared adequately through coughing, invade lung tissue, and fail to be eradicated by the patient's immune system. Potential risk factors include dental disease, poor oral hygiene, dysphagia, a weak cough reflex, a variety of medications, and factors contributing to an inadequate immune response (e.g., poor nutrition, lack of sleep, inadequate physical activity, and exposure to toxins like alcohol or cigarette smoke). Addressing all of these factors is more likely to result in a full recovery with fewer recurrences than simply giving antibiotics. Particularly when facing complex and serious challenges, it is almost always best to broaden the history before ordering more tests and treatments.

Chapter 3

Supporting Personal Growth and Development

"Our only purpose in life is growth."
—Elisabeth Kübler-Ross

"The earth is not a resting place. Man has elected to fight, not necessarily for himself, but for a process of emotional, intellectual, and ethical growth that goes on forever. To grow in the midst of dangers is the fate of the human race, because it is the law of the spirit."
—René Dubos

WHEN I WAS STILL TEACHING, I often asked medical students and residents, "Aside from differences in the subject matter, how is being a doctor different from being an auto mechanic?" They rarely came up with a plausible answer. But I was persistent. I gave them the obvious hint: "How are people different from cars?" That generated several predictable responses, such as "People have emotions," "People don't always cooperate," and, most disturbingly, "People can sue you."

Only occasionally did a student or resident respond that, unlike cars, people have aspirations. We are able to grow and develop physically, psychologically, and spiritually in response to interactions we have with others and our environment. For humans, achieving good health always involves personal growth and development.

To be fair, some auto mechanics develop relationships of a sort with some cars and with their drivers, and some mechanics are goal-oriented. In fact, some cars — think race cars, for example — grow and develop over time, but they are passive recipients of the actions taken by the mechanic. They are not actively involved. The goals and strategies are determined by the owner and mechanic, not the car.

While we normally think of growth and development as primarily a childhood concern, it is actually a lifelong process with at least two components: 1) achievement of major developmental tasks, and 2) the ongoing process of becoming more resilient, adaptable, and capable of handling challenges. Goal-oriented care takes both of these components into consideration for every patient, at every age, across time.

Developmental Tasks

The table on the next page contains a list of the major developmental tasks and the ages at which they tend to be accomplished, as proposed by developmental psychologists Erik and Joan Erikson. Within a goal-oriented conceptual framework, these can be considered developmental goals.

Each developmental task builds upon the prior ones, which means that the earliest tasks are the most critical ones. Individuals who don't develop a sense of trust during their first two or three years of life have difficulty forming relationships and dealing with losses throughout their lives. It is therefore appropriate for pediatric care to focus heavily on this goal, and that social programs exist to ensure that all infants and toddlers experience optimal growth and development during early childhood. To some degree this happens, but more could be done.

Developmental tasks receive much less attention in adults. In fact, developmental challenges in adults are more often viewed as mental health problems (e.g., social anxiety, situational depression, and midlife crisis). Viewing optimal development throughout life as a goal encourages clinicians to take a more positive, proactive approach.

I am reminded of a 40-year-old woman and her 70-year-old mother,

Table 3.1. Developmental tasks

Typical Age Range	Developmental Task	Relevant Questions
Birth to 2 years	Trust (vs. mistrust) Hope	Can I trust the world and especially the people in it?
2 to 4 years	Autonomy (vs. shame and doubt) Will	Is it OK to be me?
4 to 5 years	Initiative (vs. guilt) Purpose	Is it OK for me to do, move, and act?
5 to 12 years	Industry (vs. inferiority) Competence	Can I make it in the world?
13 to 19 years	Identity (vs. role confusion/ uncertainty Fidelity	Who am I? Who can I become?
20 to 24 years	Intimacy (vs. isolation) Love	Can I love?
25 to 64 years	Generativity (vs. stagnation) Care	Can I make my life count?
65 years to death	Ego integrity (vs. despair) Wisdom	Is it OK to have been me?

both patients of mine, the mother for more than 25 years. Since the death of her father while a teenager, the daughter had lived at home with her mother. Whenever she tried to become more independent — get a job, go on dates, etc. — the mother's many symptoms — headaches, dizziness, stomach pain, fatigue — became worse. Once I began taking care of the daughter, the situation became clearer to me.

I began to spend time at each visit teaching each of them how to contribute to the other's psychological growth. By focusing on personal development as a goal, I was able to help the daughter find the courage to get a job, move out, and get married (the identity and intimacy tasks) and the mother to proudly let her (the generativity and ego identity tasks). Those changes occurred over a two-year period of time. Individual visits, however, were not significantly longer than average.

Self-Determination Theory

Life's challenges create opportunities for physical, psychological, and spiritual growth. Health care professionals therefore have many opportunities to help patients view health events more optimistically.

Self-Determination Theory (*https://selfdeterminationtheory.org*) provides the theoretical underpinnings of goal-oriented health care. Proposed by Edward Deci and Richard Ryan, psychologists at the University of Rochester, the theory hypothesizes that there are three fundamental requirements for psychological health: relatedness, autonomy, and competence. That is, in addition to the biological requirements for life, human beings need to feel connected to others, feel free to make choices, and believe they are able to achieve outcomes important to them. When those psychological needs are not met, personal growth and development are difficult. The implications of these principles are explained in laymen's language in a book by Daniel Pink called *Drive: The Surprising Truth about What Motivates Us.*

A goal-oriented approach to health care supports all three psychological needs. Goal setting and strategic planning foster a longitudinal collaborative relationship between doctors and patients in which patients are free and encouraged to participate in decision-making. The assumption that it is possible to set and achieve goals builds both confidence and competence. Because physical abnormalities inevitably increase as we get older, problem-oriented care promotes a negative view of aging. However, personal growth and development continue to be goals throughout life and may be facilitated by the experience of loss. In fact, some have argued that it is impossible to experience optimal growth and development without facing significant challenges.

Knowledge and Skills

A rehabilitation specialist once told me, "You have to *learn* to live with a chronic illness." Successfully facing health challenges requires learning new information and skills. It should therefore not be surprising that the components of adaptability and resilience identified by experts in adult education apply equally well to health and health care. They include the knowledge and skills required to: 1) maintain and improve health; 2) become integrated within a helpful social network; and 3) develop the habits of self-assessment, reflection, goal-setting, and self-directed learning. Clinicians have many opportunities to help patients acquire the knowledge and skills required to achieve those objectives.

Physical Resilience

The most obvious example of our potential for increasing physical resilience is the immune system, which becomes more effective as we encounter germs, toxins, and cancer cells. That suggests that, for the most part, we should allow non-lethal exposures to occur. There is reasonable evidence that children raised in ultra-clean households are more likely to develop allergies, including asthma, and there is now evidence that early exposure to peanuts prevents later development of peanut allergies. Exposure to the viruses and bacteria from natural infection or immunization increases our ability to resist or limit the severity of future infections.

Actually, most systems of the body can become more resilient over time. The musculoskeletal system can become stronger as a result of strengthening exercises and more flexible with stretching. The cardio-respiratory system becomes more resilient in response to aerobic physical activity. Balance improves with balance exercises like Tai Chi. Cognition improves with use. Developing these systems beyond the capacities required for ordinary activities can enhance performance and provide the reserve capacity needed to face physical challenges, such as serious illness.

Growth and Development as a Health Goal

Personal growth and development can be assumed to be a goal for all patients. Even when it isn't the primary focus, growth and development impacts the other health goals. The lifespan orientation of goal-oriented care encourages physicians and patients to view every health event as an opportunity for both the patient and physician to become more knowledgeable and resilient.

Chapter 4

A Good Death

"Death is a process to be lived, not a problem to be solved. Yet literally every clinician my wife and I have interacted with is more afraid of death than we are; they focus on solving the problems of our illness with little awareness of how we want to live our lives."
—Stuart Farber, MD, a family physician shortly before his death

The enemy is not death. The enemy is inhumanity.
—D.G. Benfield, pediatrician, Akron, Ohio (paraphrased)

Dying Well

DISCUSSIONS ABOUT DEATH AND DYING rarely occur during routine physician-patient encounters. When they do, it is usually in the context of a life-threatening illness, typically in the hospital, long after every treatment approach has failed, and death is imminent. This is because, in problem-oriented care, death represents defeat. When a person dies, it represents a failure of medical care.

That perspective makes it difficult for physicians, patients, and families to have frank and open conversations about how and where they would like to die. It also leads to unwanted and unwarranted interventions to try to keep people alive to the too often bitter end. Some physicians have argued that they would spend more time discussing death and dying if they were paid for the time required to do so. However, after Medicare authorized payment for conversations about end-of-life preferences, a poll of 736 physicians conducted by three large non-profit organizations found that only 14% of them had ever billed for this service. A quick and dirty audit of health information exchange data from Oklahoma in 2013 suggested that advance directives were documented in fewer than 10% of patient records.

Since we will all die at some point, it makes sense to do what we can to ensure that the circumstances surrounding our deaths conform to our personal values and preferences. One of the goals of health and health care is therefore to increase the probability of a good death. Conversations regarding end-of-life preferences should begin early in adulthood, be updated yearly, and be revisited through the dying process.

The National Academy of Medicine (NAM) has defined a good death as "one that is free from avoidable distress and suffering, for patients, family, and caregivers; in general accord with the patients' and families' wishes; and reasonably consistent with clinical, cultural, and ethical standards." Medical ethicists E. J. and L. L. Emanuel have proposed six categories of modifiable factors that can contribute to the quality of the dying process: 1) physical symptoms, 2) psychological and other mental factors, 3) economic and caregiving needs, 4) social relationships and support, 5) spiritual beliefs, and 6) hopes and expectations. The relative importance of these factors varies a great deal from person to person and situation to situation.

Before I discuss ways to help people prepare for a good death, it is important to take a step back and consider how most people die and how well we can predict life expectancy.

Trajectories of Dying

The NAM introduced the concept of "trajectories of dying" as a way to conceptualize the experience of illness and dying. Joanne Lynn, palliative care researcher, used that framework to define the most common paths taken by individuals during the final stages of life. They include: Sudden Death, Terminal Illness, Major Organ Failure, and Frailty. A fifth trajectory, Catastrophic Event, has subsequently been added. When advising patients about end-of-life challenges, it is often important to consider and discuss the trajectory they appear to be on.

The sudden death and catastrophic event trajectories are self-evident. The other three are shown below.

Terminal Illness

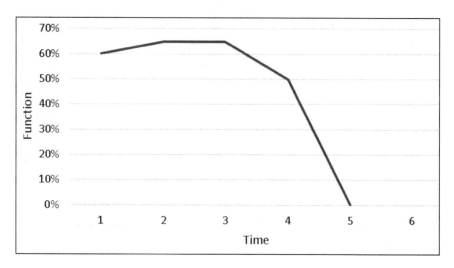

Organ Failure

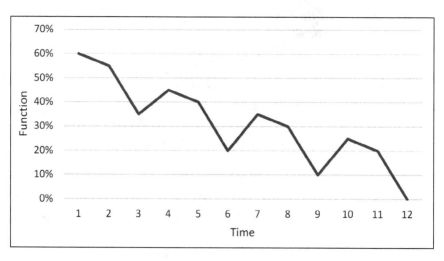

Debility/Failure to Thrive

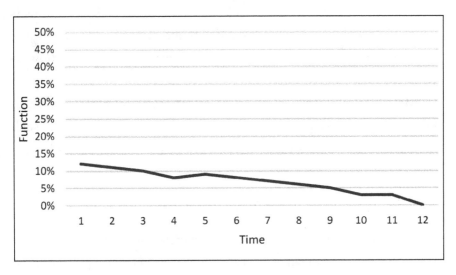

Identifying the trajectory of a patient's final years of life can be helpful when estimating life expectancy and the functional challenges ahead.

Prognosis

While physicians are notoriously inaccurate prognosticators, it is still important to consider estimated life expectancy when discussing end-of-life decisions.

I recall a 57-year-old man who had been admitted to the hospital for an exacerbation of his congestive heart failure. He had edema to his nipples and a left ventricular ejection fraction of around 15%, the result of years of alcohol and cocaine abuse. This was his fourth admission that year for the same problem, and each time diuresis had temporarily resolved his symptoms.

After reviewing his history and evaluating him, I told him he was unlikely to live much longer without a heart transplant, but he would not be considered for a transplant unless he could stop using alcohol and cocaine for at least six months and convince the transplant team that he wouldn't use them again. His response was both shocking and an indictment of our health care system. He said, "You know, Doc, I

figured I wouldn't live past 75, and that will be long enough for me."
When I said, "I think you'll be lucky to live to 59," he said, "So this is
serious!" I doubt he stopped using drugs and alcohol and had a transplant, but at least he was able to think more accurately about how to
spend the little time he had left.

My experience agrees with research that suggests patients are much
more willing to talk about death than most physicians, and that such
discussions can make a difference when decisions must be made near
the end of life.

Advance Directives

Patients who have discussed end-of-life preferences with their primary
care physicians well ahead of their deaths are less likely to be hospitalized
and less likely to undergo unwanted and unnecessary treatments during
their last 30 days of life. Even more helpful are the discussions patients
have with family members and potential surrogate decision-makers.

Some end-of-life preferences can be expressed on standard legal
forms. All 50 states now provide the opportunity for individuals living
there to complete some sort of advance directive for health care. These
documents are sometimes called "living wills." They are posted on the
website of each Secretary of State. Since we don't know when death will
come, every adult should strongly consider completing one of these documents. While advance directives tend to be associated with the elderly,
history suggests they are actually more important for younger adults, in
whom end-of-life decisions are more likely to create controversy. Notable
examples include the cases of Karen Ann Quinlan and Terri Schiavo.

Karen Ann Quinlan was 21 years old in 1975 when she took a combination of a painkiller, an anti-anxiety drug, and alcohol, experienced
hypoxemia, and lapsed into a persistent coma. Despite her parents'
request, doctors refused to take her off of the respirator. The ensuing
legal battle resulted in new regulations requiring ethics committees in
all hospitals, among other things.

Terri Schiavo was 26 when she had a cardiac arrest at her home in Florida, possibly caused by a low potassium level resulting from bulimia. Although she was successfully resuscitated by paramedics, she suffered severe brain damage and became totally dependent, requiring a feeding tube for nutrition. Schiavo's husband and legal guardian believed that she would not want to be kept alive in that condition and requested that her feeding tube be removed, but her parents argued that she always had a strong will to live and would want life support continued.

While the legal battle raged, health care professionals attempted speech and physical therapy and various experimental therapies, hoping to return Schiavo to a state of awareness, without success. Finally, after 15 years of bitter legal and eventually political strife, the feeding tube was removed, and she was allowed to die. Neither Karen Ann Quinlan nor Terri Schiavo had completed an advance directive. Had they done so, it would have made life much easier for their families and, to the degree they were aware of their own discomfort, for them.

Living wills pose several challenges for physicians. Because they are not often linked electronically to health records, they must be scanned, which makes them somewhat less accessible. Most electronic health records (EHRs) do have a place to document their existence and basic content, but that requires additional documentation. They are most often needed in the emergency room or hospital setting, but processes for transferring the information from office to hospital are still inadequate, particularly when they are needed after hours or on weekends. In addition, the conditions under which they typically apply -- imminent death or persistent coma -- occur in a small minority of the situations in which difficult decisions must be made. While designation of a surrogate decision-maker tends to be the most helpful component of legal directives, too often the designated decision-maker has been inadequately prepared for the role.

All states also allow individuals to create a Durable Power of Attorney for Health Care (DPOA-HC), in which they can specify who should make health care decisions for them if they are no longer able to speak for themselves. Unlike a regular power of attorney, a DPOA-HC only takes effect after the individual has been found to be incompetent to make decisions. Since every DPOA-HC is somewhat different, physicians must actually see and read the document to determine what types of decisions are covered, and, in particular, whether health care decisions are included.

Federal law requires that health care providers who accept Medicare or Medicaid must inform patients of their right to accept or refuse medical or surgical treatment and the right to execute an "advance directive." Patients must be asked whether they have an advance directive. If the answer is "no," however, there is no requirement to ask if they would like to have help completing one. If the answer is "yes," there is no requirement that they be asked to provide a copy of their directive to be put into their medical record. Practices and hospital admissions offices should, of course, ask those additional questions anyway.

A goal-oriented approach makes it much more likely that every competent patient will complete all of the advance directive documents available in their state as early in their adult life as possible. Copies would be kept in all pertinent medical records, by all potential family decision-makers, and in a folder attached to their refrigerators for emergency personnel to review.

Formal advance directives should be supplemented with information obtained during patient encounters and from pre-visit questionnaires. Patients should be encouraged to tell potential surrogate decision-makers about conditions they would consider worse than death and their values and preferences regarding end-of-life care.

Conditions Worse Than Death

While staying alive is an important goal for most people, most of us can think of conditions under which death would be a blessing. Over a ten-year period, my partners and I asked every new patient seen in our geriatric practice to state which was more important to them: length of life or quality of life. All patients were at least 65 years old and their average age was 78. Eighty-two percent said that quality of life was more important.

When we took a deeper look at their answers, we found something interesting. Those who chose "length of life" over "quality of life" were more likely to be disabled. That seemed counterintuitive. Why would people with disabilities be more likely to want to stay alive? In fact, the same phenomenon has been seen in longitudinal studies. As subjects became more disabled, they tended to change their preference from quality to length of life. The most likely explanation is that when we are doing well, we can't imagine being able to enjoy life with a serious disability. However, when disabilities inevitably occur, we discover that we can tolerate them better than we had imagined, and we become aware that life is nearly always better than the alternative.

We also asked patients, "What conditions, if permanent, would you consider to be worse than death?" We gave them a list of options (shown in the table below). To be sure they understood, we also posed the question in another way: "If you were in the condition in question, it was going to be permanent, and you then developed pneumonia, would you want us to give you antibiotics?" The proportions of people viewing each condition as worse than death are shown below:

Table 4.1. Conditions considered worse than death

Condition	% Rating Worse Than Death
Unable to live alone	6%
Living in a nursing home	15%
Unable to make decisions for myself	21%
Painful terminal illness	36%
Unable to recognize family members	40%
Permanent coma	85%

When we looked for personal characteristics that might predict their opinion, we couldn't find any. Age, race, marital status, educational attainment, religion, and income were all poor predictors. That means that the point at which survival would no longer be a goal must be elicited from each person. And because people often change their minds, that conversation must be repeated periodically, particularly after significant changes in functional status.

Mrs. Lively was 75 years old when her daughter brought her to see me with concerns about her mother's short-term memory loss. Both agreed that her memory was worsening. Cognitive testing confirmed the problem with short-term memory, but it also showed that her judgment and decision-making abilities were still intact. We discussed the probability that her thinking difficulties were likely to get worse over time, and I asked Mrs. Lively if there would be a point at which she would no longer want her life to be prolonged. She said that if she was unable to recognize family members she would prefer to die.

As it turned out, Mrs. Lively' s condition did progress, and about two years after our first encounter her daughter called to tell me she could no longer recognize her and reminded me of our earlier discussion. After discussing and assuring the agreement of all of her caregivers, we stopped her life-prolonging medications, and she died a few weeks later. Documentation of her wishes and engagement of her daughter and the nursing home staff significantly reduced the risk of liability claims.

Values Pertaining to End-of-Life Care

In that same pre-enrollment questionnaire, we asked patients to choose, from a list of 14 end-of-life values, the three they considered most important. The items were derived from the Values History developed by David Doukas and Laurence McCullough. Their choices are shown in Table 4.2.

Table 4.2. Percentages of patients who included each value among their top three

Value	% Ranking It Among Top Three
Thinking clearly	64%
Not being a burden to family	45%
Avoiding unnecessary pain and suffering	37%
Maintaining good relationships with family	28%
Maintaining dignity until death	28%
Making own decisions	23%
Being treated with respect	17%
Feeling safe and secure	16%
Leaving good memories	15%
Being comfortable when dying	9%
Being with loved ones at death	7%
Having religious beliefs respected	7%
Contributing to medical research	4%
Having my body respected after death	0%

Those results correspond well to my clinical experience, and they suggest the kind of discussions that are often important during the dying process. Because of the concern about being a burden, these discussions are particularly helpful when family caregivers can be involved.

Trade-Offs

Just as patients must weigh the relative importance of survival and quality of life goals, there are trade-offs to be considered when balancing survival and a good death. The most obvious example involves treatment of incurable cancers. Chemotherapy and radiation therapy can prolong life, but the adverse effects often make that additional life and the process of dying less than ideal.

Atul Gawande, in his book *Being Mortal*, does a wonderful job explaining these trade-offs and suggesting ways to address them. For example, he suggests that people who are dying should consider four questions: 1) What is your understanding of the situation and its potential outcomes? 2) What are your fears and hopes? 3) What trade-offs are you willing and unwilling to make? and 4) What course of action best serves this understanding?

When asked how they would prefer to die, most people say, "in my sleep." Death during sleep is most likely to result from myocardial ischemia or infarction, a stroke, or some other cardiovascular event. Measures to reduce the risk of heart attacks and strokes therefore reduce the likelihood of our preferred type of death. Given that fact, there is often a point when lowering blood pressure and cholesterol levels are more likely to reduce the probability of a good death than to reduce premature death and disability.

Death and dying have a profound impact on family members. A particularly interesting case, about which I was informally consulted, involved a couple who had been married for 50 years. The husband tended to avoid doctors until he was seriously ill. Clinic visits almost always resulted in hospitalizations. He had survived a series of heart attacks and strokes but was still able to function as the local director of the American Association of Retired Persons (AARP).

His wife, on the other hand, saw her family physician nearly every other week. Her symptoms, which varied from visit to visit, always seemed to resolve with time and reassurance. When she developed hematuria, however, she was advised to have additional tests. When she asked what the tests might reveal, her physician mentioned the possibility of cancer. At that point she stated emphatically that she didn't want the tests. When asked why, she began to cry, saying, "I've been so afraid that my husband would die and leave me all alone. You know he has almost died several times already. My greatest hope is that I will die first. If I have cancer, that would be a blessing! Let's not do the tests and hope that's what it is."

That, of course, led to a long-overdue discussion with her physician, which might have prevented many of her previous symptoms and medical visits. He encouraged her to talk with her husband. She did eventually agree to further testing, which showed no signs of cancer.

Final Thoughts

When the absence of health problems is the goal, death represents a failure of medical care, a defeat in the war against disease. When there are no more abnormalities to correct, physicians are often at a loss as to what to do. Patients may feel abandoned. The failure of the problem-oriented model to comfortably accommodate death and dying resulted in the emergence of the field of palliative care and the creation of hospice services.

Within a goal-oriented framework, death is recognized to be an inevitable part of life. Maintaining the highest possible quality of life, experiencing personal growth and development, and preparing for a good death are goals throughout life. There is no point at which the physician's role becomes unclear, and there is no need for a separate palliative care system. However, the specialized knowledge and skills of those who have subspecialized in palliative care will be invaluable.

Chapter 5

Children, Parents, and Caregivers, Families, and Communities

"It's easier to build strong children than to repair broken men."
—Frederick Douglass

"More than ever before, there is a global understanding that long-term social, economic, and environmental development would be impossible without healthy families, communities, and countries."
—Gro Harlem Brundtland

Prevention of Premature Death in Children

RECOGNIZE THAT MY TENDENCY as a geriatrician is to focus on adults. Goal-oriented care is, in my opinion, essential for the provision of person-centered care for complex and older patients, but applies equally well to all patients, including children. The obvious differences include the essential role of parents, the reduced likelihood of death and disability, and the increased importance of growth and development.

While premature death is less likely to occur during childhood, when it does happen, the number of years of potential life lost is large. In infants and toddlers, it is important to address risk factors for sudden infant death syndrome, injuries, poisoning, preventable infections and environmental risk factors (e.g., second-hand cigarette smoke), and adverse childhood events. In older children, encouragement of physical activity and school performance become important, and, in teenagers, the focus shifts to risky behaviors and irrevocable mistakes like experimenting with addictive substances, driving while impaired, contributing to a pregnancy, acquiring a chronic sexually transmitted disease, and dropping out of school.

The ten most frequent causes of death during childhood are shown in Table 5.1. Though still at the top of the list, deaths from motor vehicle accidents have been reduced with seatbelt and child car seat practices. Similar reductions could probably be seen in firearm-related deaths if safety measures are similarly implemented and enforced. A goal-oriented approach makes it easier to explain to parents why firearm safety is discussed during well-child exams. It is because one of our goals is to prevent premature death, and firearm accidents are the second leading cause of death in children.

Table 5.1. Ten most frequent causes of death in children

Cause of Death	% of Deaths
Motor vehicle accidents	20%
Firearm-related	15.4%
Cancer	9.1%
Suffocation	7.0%
Drowning	4.9%
Poisoning	4.8%
Congenital Abnormalities	4.8%
Heart Disease	2.9%
Fire/Burns	1.7%
Chronic lower respiratory disease	1.3%

Adrian M. was a 12-year-old African American boy being raised by a single mother. They lived below the median income in a high-crime, urban neighborhood, and his mother kept a loaded, unlocked pistol in her bedroom. Adrian ate a high fat, sugar, and sodium-containing diet, with relatively few fruits and vegetables. His body mass index was in the 65th percentile. He was not very active physically, choosing to stay inside and watch television. He did sometimes ride a bicycle without a helmet. There was a family history of hypertension, diabetes mellitus type 2, and stroke. He was up-to-date on his immunizations.

Based upon a validated risk prediction algorithm developed by a colleague, Dr. Zsolt Nagykaldi, at the University of Oklahoma, Adrian was projected to live to age 67. If his mother implemented all of the preventive measures indicated for him, the algorithm predicted that he could gain an additional 4.2 years of life. The three most impactful preventive measures and their predicted impacts on life expectancy are shown below. The predictive model did include the option of moving to a safer neighborhood, though I suspect that might have an even larger effect than the measures listed.

Table 5.2. Preventive measures indicated for Adrian
and their predicted impact

Preventive measure	Years of Life Gained
Increased physical activity to recommended level	2.5
Firearm safety measures	1.2
Halthier dier	0.5
All other preventive measures	<0.1

As with adults, some children have health challenges that are associated with predictable causes of early death and disability, and, as with complex adults, a goal-oriented approach can focus attention on the most important risk factors. Obvious examples are inherited disorders of metabolism, other genetic syndromes, and birth defects.

Quality of Life in Children

Quality of life is as important for children as for adults. Because it is more heavily influenced by family and peers, however, it requires a somewhat different approach. Substituted judgment requires parents to view their children as unique individuals, separate from themselves and their own aspirations. Discovery of each child's unique interests and skills requires that they have the freedom and opportunity to explore as many activities as possible.

When I was a child, after school my friends, siblings, and I played softball and tag football, climbed trees, built forts, caught frogs and turtles, collected feathers, traded baseball cards, and explored the woods near our house. I am told the dangers of injury and abduction were higher then than now, but no one seemed to be worried about those things. As a family, we went on road trips, camped, fished, hiked, played board games, and assembled puzzles. My mother taught us "modern math" during the summers and helped me put together a cat skeleton when I was home with the measles. I was a Cub Scout and then a Boy Scout. We went to Sunday school fairly regularly or walked in the woods. I played clarinet and later oboe in the band. We watched some television, but there was no need to put limits on our screen time because there were so many other things to do.

Today, for a host of reasons, many children are more closely watched and more assiduously protected. Activities tend to be more structured and supervised. There is a greater emphasis on competition. Our daughter loved gymnastics, but at the age of 11, she was required to practice three to four hours a day, which occupied nearly all of her free time. My son had band practices on weekends, holidays, and during the summer. Some children are involved in way too many activities, while others have limited opportunities to participate. Physicians can often help parents remember that the goal is to help their children grow up to be happy, healthy, independent adults.

Decision-making for children with developmental disabilities or major environmental, social, or behavioral difficulties can be particularly challenging. A goal-oriented approach is especially valuable just as it is for complex adult patients, and the questions are similar: "What is a typical day like? What daily activities are most difficult? What does the child seem to enjoy? What do you think they would like to achieve next?" As with adults, rehabilitation therapists and other allied health professionals can be invaluable.

Growth and Development During Childhood

A great deal of attention is already paid to growth and development during childhood, which is appropriate given the importance of the foundational developmental stages and the rapidity of the changes that occur during this period of life. The goal-oriented approach focuses on strategies to ensure achievement rather than identification of delays and failures to reach milestones. To a significant degree, pediatricians have already adopted this approach.

A Good Death

Discussing death with the parents of children at high risk of dying can be particularly difficult. Experts suggest helping families prepare for both best and worst-case scenarios and then developing an emergency care plan that includes resuscitation preferences and other family priorities.

Promoting and Maintaining Family Health and Harmony

When the specialty of Family Medicine was established, some of its founding fathers believed that the focus of care should be on families rather than individuals, thus the name. Given the strong influence of families on health, the idea had strong theoretical merit. However, its application proved to be extremely difficult. Beyond questions about who should be counted as family, there were ethical concerns (e.g. confidentiality and autonomy) that were never fully resolved. As a result, most primary care physicians believe that their contractual obligation is with individual patients, not families. Improving family health and stability are unquestionably important objectives along the path toward the survival, quality of life, growth and development, and good death goals of individual patients.

The same principle applies to caregivers of people with disabilities. There is no question that caregiver health and well-being are critically important to those for whom they provide care, and so physicians should promote caregiver health as a way to help their patients achieve their goals.

Communities

The health of patients and their families is heavily dependent upon the health of the communities in which they live. Investment in the health of individual patients therefore compels physicians to do what we can to address the social and environmental determinants of health. Focusing on patient goals inevitably reveals common sets of obstacles and challenges, which we can often help to address by serving on community boards and committees or by simply speaking out when opportunities arise. Some of those obstacles and challenges will be easily addressed, a new walking path, removing soft drink machines from schools. Some will involve inequities and prejudices deeply rooted in our history and politics.

Because we have accepted responsibility for helping patients achieve their personal health goals, we have agreed to help them with the obstacles and challenges they face. In a speech to a group of medical students entitled "To Isaiah," later published in the *Journal of the*

American Medical Association in 2020, Donald Berwick, former Director of the Centers for Medicare and Medicaid Services wrote, "Now you don your white coats, and you enter a career of privilege. Society gives you rights and license it gives to no one else, in return for which you promise to put the interests of those for whom you care ahead of your own. That promise and that obligation give you voice in public discourse simply because of the oath you have sworn. Use that voice. If you do not speak, who will."

Section 2

Obstacles and Challenges

W HEN I EXPLAIN GOAL-ORIENTED CARE to physicians, a typical first response is, "That's what we do." Once I've convinced them that it isn't, their response is, "It isn't
possible."

By the way, it isn't hard to convince doctors that they aren't practicing goal-oriented care. All I have to do is show them their rates of
delivery of high impact preventive services, the lack of recorded information about their patients' daily activities, and their rates of documentation of advance directives.

In fairness, it is difficult to fully implement goal-oriented care. To
do so, physicians will need additional training, a different record-keep-
ing system, more advanced decision-support tools, and a different billing process. Delivering goal-oriented care will also require a different
kind of primary care team and better information about how to help
patients achieve their goals. Gathering that information will require
new research methods.

However, I know that it is possible to apply many of the principles of goal-oriented care. It is, first and foremost, a mindset, a different way of thinking. Once you have adopted that mindset, goal-oriented care can be provided even within a problem-oriented health care system. In this section of the book I will discuss some of the major obstacles and how we can begin to overcome and eventually eliminate them.

Chapter 6

Electronic Health Records (EHRs)

"It has become appallingly clear that technology has exceeded our humanity."
—Albert Einstein

"Tellingly, the more advanced the EHR; for example, systems that offer reminders, alerts, and messaging capability, the greater the unhappiness."
—Robert Wachter, MD

I RECENTLY SCHEDULED AN APPOINTMENT with my primary care physician. In preparation for the visit, I was asked to answer a number of questions online using the practice's electronic portal. There were the usual questions about my current and past medical problems, surgical procedures, and family medical history. On the final page of the questionnaire there was a single question about me, the person. It asked, "Please tell us who lives with you and any other pertinent information about yourself." I wrote, "I live with my wife, Sandy, and my golden retriever, Lily. I . . ." At that point I ran out of space, so I deleted the "I."

There were no questions about important and meaningful life activities, advance directives, resources, limitations, or personal values. I was curious to see how the tidbit of personal information I was able to provide was handled in my medical record, so I went back online to find it. It was gone. I'm sure it's in there somewhere, but it was neither visible nor modifiable by me.

A Brief History of Medical Records

For the first half of the twentieth century, the structure and content of medical records were determined by the physicians who created them, which was fine since they were the only ones who saw them. They were handwritten and often illegible to everyone other than their creators. Because the notes were succinct, entire records could be kept on several index cards stapled together. A typical visit note looked like this:

Strep throat. Pen VK 250mg QID X 10 days.

By the time I entered medical school in 1970, records were kept in manila folders containing separate sections for comprehensive evaluations, hospital discharge summaries, test results, and progress notes. Comprehensive exams and hospital admission evaluations typically included a history of present illnesses, past medical history, social history, family medical history, review of systems, physical examination, assessments, and plans. Interim visit notes were mostly short phrases without subheadings, documenting new findings and actions taken.

In 1964, Lawrence Weed, a general internist from Vermont, in anticipation of computerization, suggested a new documentation method that he called the "problem-oriented medical record." He recommended that the first section contain a robust "patient profile" describing the patient as a person. He proposed that the history of present illness and every progress note be composed of separate paragraphs for each medical problem in SOAP (subjective, objective, assessment, plan) format. That would allow the clinician to easily trace the history of individual problems over time. Finally, he suggested that every record include a list of all of the active health problems identified in that individual, the "problem list." Weed's ideas began to take hold in the early 1970's, and most of them eventually were adopted by clinicians, insurance companies, and electronic health records vendors.

The problem-oriented medical record was accepted because it was a better representation of the way physicians had learned to think. It reflected the rapid advancement of the science of diseases and their treatment. Unfortunately, some of Weed's best ideas, such as placing a personal description of the patient at the beginning of the record and orienting progress notes in such a way that problems could be more easily tracked over time, were largely ignored. Weed went on to develop an electronic medical record system that linked problems to published evidence -- the Problem-Knowledge Coupler -- but that idea never caught on.

Despite all of the touted benefits of computerization, the health care system was slow to embrace and adopt computer technologies. EHRs have been available since the 1970s, but, as recently as ten years ago, they were used by a small minority of physicians and hospitals. In an all-out effort to improve coordination of care and reduce costs, the federal government, during the Obama administration, made EHR implementation a priority. Financial incentives were paid to physicians and hospitals through both Medicare and Medicaid to help with the cost of conversion from paper to electronic records. Health information technology regional extension centers (HIT-RECs) were established to help practices with implementation. As of January 2015, all doctors had to be using electronic medical records to avoid financial penalties, and most have done so.

The Evolving Purpose of Medical Records

Prior to 1985, the main purpose of medical records was to document clinical information useful for patient care. Payment for medical services was based on the concept of "customary, prevailing, and reasonable rates," as determined by the physician, and based largely on time spent with the patient. As the number of medical malpractice lawsuits increased during the second half of the twentieth century, better documentation became necessary, and notes became longer, but their primary purpose remained: to support clinical care.

Of course, some physicians overcharged, others complained, and Medicare felt compelled to tighten its billing and reimbursement criteria. Since 1985, several significant changes have been made in the way

the value of physicians' services is calculated. Medicaid and private insurance companies have, for the most part, followed suit. Those
changes required more detailed documentation, so detailed in fact that
many physicians chose to accept lower fees rather than spend the time
to learn and follow the new requirements.

The challenge presented by the new billing rules provided a window
of opportunity for the developers of EHRs. Physicians otherwise reluctant to purchase expensive electronic record systems could be convinced
that the records would pay for themselves by facilitating the documentation required for higher reimbursement rates. That marketing strategy
resulted in the development of EHRs designed primarily for the opti-
mization of billing and reimbursement, not patient care.

The ability to generate preprogrammed verbiage by clicking buttons
has resulted in notes so long and redundant that, once created, they are
hardly ever read again by anyone. And despite the promise of greater
efficiency and higher reimbursement rates, most primary care physicians have found that the time spent on documentation has actually increased. Many have had to reduce the number of patients they see each
day, and they still have to work through lunch and into the evening
just to complete their records. Both physicians and patients complain
that the computer interferes with person-to-person interactions during
visits.

Electronic Medical Records Systems
and Goal-Oriented Care

The problem-oriented structure of EHRs is a significant barrier to
the adoption and implementation of goal-oriented care. Only a few
EHRs display any sort of personal information on the opening page.
In most cases, that information is buried in the Social History section,
accessible only by clicking several buttons. The most prominent sections of most records are the Problem List and the Medication List,
which tend to drive the agenda for non-acute care visits. Visit notes are,

for the most part, created by clicking boxes in pre-coded problem-oriented templates. A Disposition section requires labeling and coding each concern dealt with at the visit.

Aside from the problem list, there is no one place where risk factors for premature death can be documented. While most EHRs generate reminders of preventive services for which patients are eligible, none are able to prioritize them by projected impact on life extension or prevention of disability. There is no convenient and appropriate place to document important and meaningful life activities. Only pediatric records include forms on which to document personal growth and development, and they generally include just the standard developmental milestones. Most systems have a section in which to indicate whether the patient has an advance directive, but the documents themselves must usually be scanned into the record. There is no designated place to record conditions under which individual patients would no longer wish to be kept alive and preferences for end-of-life care.

Electronic health records are perhaps the greatest impediment to full implementation of goal-oriented care because they are so rigidly problem-oriented and so expensive to replace.

A Way Forward

One solution would be to establish a common, generic, open-access database designed to accept, categorize, and link the full range of relevant patient information from all authorized sources (i.e., clinicians, hospitals, laboratories, imaging facilities, pharmacists, dentists, rehabilitation therapists, and patients). Health care providers could access this universal database through any of a variety of user interfaces, each designed for a specific purpose and type of user. Private vendors could compete to build the most user-friendly interfaces for clinicians, patients, quality monitors, billing staff, and insurance companies.

A goal-oriented interface could organize relevant information into the four major goal domains. For example, risk factors would populate algorithms for prioritizating preventive strategies. Information relevant to valued life activities would be aggregated in a quality of life section. Similarly, there would be sections for personal growth and development and end-of-life planning. Each section would include timelines on which to track and view progress and reminders of potentially helpful strategies. Additional features might include clinical pathways for common objectives like smoking cessation and links to community and other resources.

Meanwhile

Although current EHRs don't support goal-oriented care, they don't prevent it. Just as physicians have learned to satisfy coding and billing requirements which, more often than not, don't reflect what actually goes on during clinical encounters, it is possible to circumvent the obstacles created by EHRs.

The problem list can be reconceptualized as a list of risk factors, and current disease-based registries can be combined into single preventive service registries that include primary, secondary, and tertiary preventive services. Most record systems have templates for functional assessments. These could be reconfigured to capture important and meaningful life activities and the objectives and strategies relevant to them. End-of life values and preferences can often be summarized in the advance directives section with reference to the date of the visit note when they were last discussed.

Hopefully someone reading this book will have the energy and ability to assemble a team to develop a goal-oriented record system before current systems collapse under the weight of the data that will surely be coming from personal monitoring devices and genetic testing.

Chapter 7

Coding and Billing

"You don't train someone for all of those years of medical school and residency, particularly people who want to help others optimize their physical and psychological health, and then have them run a claims-processing operation for insurance companies."
—Malcolm Gladwell

"The virtue-based physician could never see his patient as a 'customer,' consumer, insured life or any other commercialized, industrialized transformations of the ancient and respectable word 'patient.'"
—Edmund D. Pellegrino, MD

Reimbursement for Cognitive Services

IT HAS ALWAYS BEEN DIFFICULT for health insurance companies to figure out how much to pay clinicians for non-procedural services. How valuable is the application of knowledge, wisdom, and judgment? What about the time required to establish relationships with patients, review medical records from previous physicians, or coordinate care? What is it worth when a primary care physician convinces a patient to have a colonoscopy or helps a patient stop smoking or reduce their consumption of alcohol? Should health insurance companies reimburse practices for the time and support required for continuous quality improvement?

I vividly remember, during my first years in private practice, successfully resuscitating a man in our office and spending the next hour keeping him alive until the physicians at the hospital could take over. He had had a heart attack followed by cardiac arrest in the examination room adjacent to my office. It was a Saturday, and our newly hired staff was unfamiliar with our resuscitation equipment. When the small-town rescue squad arrived, they realized they had forgotten to bring a defibrillator and had to go back for it. The EKG monitor in their ambulance didn't work, so, during the 20-minute drive to the hospital, I conversed with the patient while feeling the pulse in his wrist. When he stopped talking and his pulse disappeared, I shocked him. That happened at least four times.

When we got to the emergency room, he was in atrial fibrillation, alert with a good blood pressure. After relating the history to the ER physician, I went directly home, exhausted and covered in vomit, sweat, and blood. My wife remembers my asking her how much she thought I should charge him. I wondered whether $100 would be too much. (Remember, this was 1979 and I was only recently out of residency.)

I saw that same man, who was not a regular patient of ours, in the office for a minor illness a year later. I don't think he remembered who I was. After all, he wasn't himself that day. I don't recall what I ended up charging him for saving his life. He didn't complain about it, and I never worried that Medicare would audit my records and make me pay them back.

In the late 1970s, insurance companies generally trusted physicians to charge appropriately, and the vast majority of us did. However, a small proportion predictably cheated. Rather than seeking out and punishing the cheaters, the federal government decided to make it more difficult for all physicians to cheat. In an attempt to tighten up the billing process in 1985, the Centers for Medicare and Medicaid Services (CMS) commissioned the development of a new value-based reimbursement system based upon a complicated formula that included the amount of physical effort, skill required, malpractice risk, and complexity involved in each patient encounter. Since no actual data existed upon which to determine the values of the new factors, the system wasn't well-accepted and didn't work very well.

The Evaluation and Management Approach

In 1992, the algorithm was modified to include documentation of physician work (questions asked, diagnoses made, treatments prescribed), practice expense (estimated as an average by a special panel of physicians), and cost of malpractice insurance (average for the specialty of the physician). The physician work component accounted for 48% of the total. It was called Evaluation and Management (E&M) coding.

E&M coding was a points-based system with points awarded for each appropriate question asked by the doctor (history taking), each part of the physical examination completed, and the complexity of the visit as determined by the number of problems managed, lab tests ordered, and prescriptions written (decision-making). The total "value" of each visit was based roughly on the number of points in each area (history, exam, decision-making), multiplied by a factor derived from number of years of training and risk of liability. While it was possible to bill based upon time spent, the reimbursement rate was typically lower than the rates for bullet point-based visits. In order to submit a bill to Medicare for any visit, at least one and no more than four diagnoses had to be listed on the billing form. Medicaid and most private insurance companies adopted the same billing method.

Aside from being more complicated and probably no more fair or accurate than previous methods, E&M coding effectively locked doctors into a problem-oriented approach. It assumed that medical care is almost entirely about diagnosing and treating medical problems. However, in my primary care geriatric practice, most visits weren't about that at all. Most involved helping patients with chronic health challenges live longer and function better. Physical examination was only occasionally helpful for purposes other than reassurance. While I was always able to come up with a list of "diagnoses" for billing purposes, that list rarely captured what actually happened during the visit. Many physicians, including me, refused to memorize the complex E&M rules and simply undercharged to avoid getting into trouble with the auditors. Others hired additional staff to calculate the correct billing codes, while still others bought electronic medical record systems that would do the calculation electronically.

Managed Care, Accountable Care Organizations, and Value-Based Purchasing

The E&M coding and billing method was created for use in a fee-for-service delivery system, which has been the predominant payment model for medical services throughout history. However, economists have pointed out that the fee-for-service approach incentivizes doctors to provide more services. They argue that fee-for-service is an important factor contributing to rising health care costs. It has also led to shorter primary care visits and more prescriptions and referrals as primary care physicians try to make their hamster wheels spin faster.

In the 1980s, many Medicaid programs and some commercial insurers instituted a radically different payment process called "managed care." In a managed care model, primary care physicians are paid a set amount of money per patient per month and are then expected to provide comprehensive and coordinated care. A certain percentage of the payments are withheld, and later paid, along with a percentage of any savings accrued, at the end of each year if the cost of care has been less than projected. Because these end-of-year payments are based upon the total cost of care for these patients, including the care provided by subspecialists and hospitals, primary care physicians are financially incentivized to reduce referrals and consultations as well as emergency room visits and hospitalizations.

Managed care puts primary care physicians in the role of "gate-keepers," a role they first welcomed but soon rejected as they found themselves trying to talk patients out of requested services, wondering if it was for financial or valid medical reasons. Despite this obvious conflict of interest, some managed care plans have survived (e.g., Kaiser Permanente and some Medicaid plans), but most were abandoned in favor of a return to fee-for-service or some combination of fee-for-service and managed care.

Passage of the Patient Protection and Affordable Care Act in 2010 established the Centers for Medicare and Medicaid Innovations (CMMI), the mission of which was to improve the quality and effectiveness of health care while reducing its cost. A number of important experiments have been conducted or are underway, all of which involve new payment models. The two approaches that appear to have gained the most traction to date are "accountable care organizations" (ACOs) and "value-based purchasing."

Value-based purchasing ties some portion of reimbursement rates for individual physicians to both cost and quality of care since "value" is defined as quality divided by cost. ACOs are essentially managed care organizations that attempt to incentivize entire systems of doctors and hospitals to reduce costs and improve quality.

By adding the quality of care component, these models attempt to reduce the impact of the conflict of interest created by tying financial gain to medical decisions. That strategy rests on the very questionable assumption that value can be fairly and accurately measured using current problem-oriented metrics. It assumes, for example, that nearly everyone with an elevated blood pressure needs, wants, and has the resources necessary to bring their blood pressure down to the same "ideal" level. It also assumes that blood pressure reduction is a reliable measure of the quality of care delivered by clinicians regardless of their patient population. But those assumptions simply aren't true.

For example, a physician with an upper middle class, well-educated suburban practice, who is really good at getting patients' blood pressure under control regardless of whether it is beneficial to them, would be credited with providing high quality care. On the other hand, a physician working in a free clinic where most patients are unable to afford medications, and many are addicted to alcohol or have serious mental illnesses, would receive lower quality scores and less reimbursement even if they had chosen to focus on the social and behavioral risk factors with greater impacts on health than elevated blood pressure.

Recognizing that a small percentage of patients account for a high percentage of health care costs, additional billing codes have been added to reimburse practices for management of complex patients. Complexity is typically defined by some combination of multiple medical problems and high utilization rates. Not surprisingly, care management strategies tend to be disease-oriented and not particularly effective at lowering costs or improving meaningful outcomes. In addition, most practices don't have the financial reserves required to invest in the additional staff and technologies needed to provide it.

Goal-oriented health care will function best in a world in which health care is viewed as a public good rather than a commodity, the assumption being that our society is stronger when we are all healthy. It seems to me that primary care, at least, should be exempted from the reimbursement schemes discussed above since greater access to primary care is associated with higher quality of care, better patient outcomes, and lower health care costs. If physician incentives were deemed necessary, they should be based upon care process measures (e.g., access, coordination, continuity, comprehensiveness, accountability) and patient-oriented outcomes (e.g., estimated life expectancy, quality of life, personal growth and development, advanced care planning, cost of care). In addition to physician reimbursement, funding should be provided for continuous quality improvement, research and development, and investment in new care processes and technologies.

Meanwhile

Primary care physicians have had to learn to adapt to billing requirements whether or not they reflect what actually happens during clinical encounters. However, the addition of problem-oriented quality measures has created new challenges for those trying to practice person-centered care. It seems to me that there are at least three ways to think about this.

First, the attempt to measure quality of care is not an intrinsically bad idea. Many have argued that quality can only be improved when it can be measured. The issue is with the measures. Instead of once again blindly adapting, this is the time to propose more appropriate quality measures for primary care, and the organizations tasked with developing measures seem willing to listen.

Second, most payers seem to understand that 100% adherence to quality measures is neither possible nor desirable. Because the disease-oriented measures are probably appropriate for helping many, if not most, patients achieve their health goals, there shouldn't be a big problem meeting most of them. Primary care physicians should insist though that there be a way to opt patients out of the denominators of measures that are inappropriate, given their circumstances.

Finally, when care is designed around patient-relevant goals, adherence ought to improve substantially. Therefore, when plan-of-care objectives include management of diseases for which measures have been established, achievement of metric targets should improve. Said another way, even though fewer patients would want or need to meet the disease-based targets, those who did would be more likely to achieve them because of better adherence to required strategies.

Chapter 8

Clinical Practice Guidelines and Quality Measures

"Whereas in times past the 'right thing' was an ethical construct enshrined in the values of the caregiving professions, it is now a particular drug, test, or strategy supported by the burgeoning medical literature."

—Richard M.J. Bohmer

"The unbridled enthusiasm for guidelines, and the unrealistic expectations about what they will accomplish, frequently betrays inexperience and unfamiliarity with their limitations and potential hazards."

—Steven H. Woolf, MD, MPH and colleagues

Clinical Practice Guidelines

IN THE LATE 1980s, STUDIES CONDUCTED by Jack Wennberg at Dartmouth, now updated regularly in *The Dartmouth Atlas of Health Care*, showed wide geographic variation in the rates of performance of a number of medical procedures. Those revelations, combined with advances in research analytic methodologies, contributed to the birth of "evidence-based medicine," defined as "the conscientious, explicit, and judicious use of current best evidence in making decisions about the care of individual patients."

By following stringent methodologic rules and advanced search strategies, researchers are now able to create relatively unbiased systematic reviews. Advanced statistical methods make it possible to combine and summarize the results of multiple clinical studies, producing "meta-analyses." Systematic reviews and meta-analyses can then be used to develop clinical practice guidelines (CPGs). The original hope and promise of CPGs was that they would reduce unnecessary tests and treatments and protect physicians from lawsuits. They were never intended to be rigid or binding. While, in many ways, they represent a step forward, there have been a number of unintended adverse consequences.

CPGs are nearly always disease-focused, and the vast majority focus on single diseases. Each is developed independently, with little attempt at harmonization across diseases, even though most people over the age of fifty have multiple chronic conditions. In a now classic paper published in *The Journal of the American Medical Association*, Cynthia Boyd and her colleagues showed that application of CPGs to a patient with five common medical problems - hypertension, osteoarthritis, osteoporosis, type 2 diabetes mellitus, and chronic obstructive lung disease - resulted in a complicated regimen of twelve different medications with multiple potential drug interactions.

Not surprisingly, CPGs contribute to disease-oriented care. Primary care physicians have learned that the best way to make sure that all CPG-based quality metrics are met is to schedule subspecialty-like visits in which single diseases are managed by protocol. Electronic health record templates make it possible for many conditions to be "managed" by non-physicians. CPG-based registries generate lists of patients due for tests or treatments. Physicians often refer to this as "cookbook medicine."

A CPG orientation can also contribute to fragmented thinking, the failure to integrate multiple pieces of information. While teaching at a local nursing home, I met a woman I will call Jane. Jane had recently been discharged from the hospital after a three-week stay during which she almost died from disturbances of her blood chemistries, kidney failure, confusion and hallucinations, anemia, and malnutrition. This admission was the longest in a series of hospitalizations over the prior year. Upon reviewing all of her hospital discharge summaries, it was clear that she had received excellent disease-oriented care. Every individual abnormality had been addressed. At the time of discharge her lab test results were as good as they were going to be.

Very little information was available from Jane's records about who she was as a person or why she became so sick again and again. However, buried within her Social History was a mention of occasional heavy alcohol use, which seemed important in view of her many clinical abnormalities. I decided, with her permission, to sit down and talk with her and her two daughters. During our conversation Jane and her daughters revealed that, over the past year or more, Jane had lived with a boyfriend who she acknowledged was an alcoholic. Her daughters reported that since she had been living with him, she had also been drinking heavily. They believed she would be unable to quit drinking as long as she was in that environment.

I looked back at her recent medical history. Nearly everything could be explained on the basis of alcohol misuse. I told Jane in the presence of her daughters that if she continued to drink heavily, she would almost certainly end up back in the hospital, and the next time she could very easily die. I emphasized the point by asking her to consider all the reasons she had for wanting to stay alive. Jane was clearly not ready to die. She reluctantly agreed that she wouldn't be able to stop drinking as long as she was living with her boyfriend. One of the daughters invited Jane to live with her, and she decided to try it, at least for a while.

Jane subsequently became my patient. She did not return to the boyfriend and was able to quit drinking. As a result, she did well for a number of years until her kidneys eventually failed, requiring dialysis. In theory, Jane might have done as well with disease-oriented care if her most important disease, alcoholism, had been identified. However, the doctors who cared for her became distracted by all of her individual problems, the ones that were more obvious because they produced abnormal laboratory test results. By focusing on the goal — prevention of premature death – I was able to prioritize her alcohol abuse and clarify the situation for her and her daughters in a way that helped the three of them develop effective strategies.

Quality Metrics

Goodhart's Law: "When a measure becomes a target, it ceases to be a good measure."
—*Charles Goodhart, economist*

Campbell's Law: "The more a metric is used, the more likely it is to corrupt the process it is intended to monitor."
—*Donald T. Campbell, psychologist*

Efforts by economists, policy makers, and insurance companies to reduce the cost of health care have included the use of CPGs to develop quality of care standards. The belief is that tying physician reimbursement to quality of care and encouraging competition by providing patients with comparative quality metrics will reduce health care costs through market-based competition. There are several problems with this approach. Most importantly, health care doesn't (and probably shouldn't) behave like other commodities, and, as stated earlier, physicians shouldn't be put in the position of deciding between their personal financial interests and the interests of their patients. For example, physicians shouldn't be financially rewarded for performing tests or prescribing treatments for patients who will probably benefit very little from them.

Quality measures derived from CPGs create the impression that all CPG recommendations should be acted upon and every person with the same condition should be treated the same way (e.g., everyone should have a blood pressure of less than 140/90). CPGs rarely quantify the average patient-relevant benefits of each recommendation, making it difficult for physicians to base their recommendations on patient goals. This conceptualization of quality resembles the approach used in factories where the objective is to assure that every widget produced is identical. Such a view is antithetical to goal-oriented care, in which the assumption is that every person is unique and should be treated differently.

Keeping blood pressure below 140/90 is more important for some people than for others, and, for some people, it is entirely irrelevant and unnecessary. The ideal blood pressure for each person is dependent upon their individual risk profile, life circumstances, and goals. Even if keeping blood pressure below 140/90 could reduce the risk of strokes, heart attacks, heart failure, and kidney damage in a particular individual, those benefits might not be worth the time, effort, anxiety, and money that could be better spent on other strategies with greater value for that person (e.g., treatment of alcoholism).

To be most useful to payers and for physician quality ratings, quality indicators must be accessible from billing information or mandatory electronic reporting. That means they must be codable. Laboratory tests like hemoglobin A1c or procedures like mammography are therefore preferred; attributes such as accessibility, continuity, coordination, and comprehensiveness not as much; and interventions like education, reassurance, encouragement, reframing, and processes like goal-setting not at all.

Finally, several studies have affirmed that, when it comes to quality metric-based reimbursement, you get what you pay for. That is, physicians learn to focus on meeting the quality standards, often neglecting other important aspects of care. There is no evidence that either positive or negative financial incentives based upon CPG-derived quality metrics improve patient outcomes or reduce health care costs. There is, however, evidence suggesting that physicians dislike it intensely and that it is a contributor to the increasing rate of burnout.

Clinical Practice Guidelines and Electronic Registries

With the development of vaccines, antibiotics, workplace safety regulations, improved treatments for developmental challenges, and other public health measures, the incidence and severity of acute health problems have been reduced. Replacing them in importance to health care professionals and their patients are chronic health challenges associated with aging, inactivity, poor diets, smoking, and environmental hazards. In an effort to help doctors move from an acute to a chronic, longitudinal care orientation, researchers led by Ed Wagner at the MacColl Center for Health Care Innovation in Seattle and Tom Bodenheimer at the University of California San Francisco developed a conceptual model, which has served as a map for improving the delivery of primary care. One component of their "Chronic Care Model," information systems, has led to the development of "registries" to manage subpopulations of patients, and this has become a standard way to meet the quality standards.

A registry electronically receives and stores information on all patients in a doctor's practice with a particular health condition (e.g., diabetes) from which various analyses and reports can be produced. The registries can be used to produce lists of patients who, for whatever reasons, have not had all guideline-recommended visits, tests, or procedures or whose conditions have not been controlled to guideline-recommended targets. Those patients can then be contacted, either by computer-generated letter, e-mail, or phone, and advised to come in to remedy the situation. Flags may also appear in the electronic medical record reminding physicians to take care of the deficiencies during visits scheduled for other reasons.

Nearly all current registries are disease-based, with a separate registry for each disease for which guidelines exist. In concept, registries make sense. Their purpose is to systematize care so that important clinical strategies are not forgotten. However, disease-specific registries reinforce problem-oriented care in at least three ways: 1) by focusing on disease-oriented strategies and metrics rather than meaningful, patient-relevant outcomes; 2) by creating subtle pressure to clean up the task list even when some tasks wouldn't otherwise be considered necessary; and 3) by shifting decision-making from doctors to office staff or automated notification systems that advise actions without considering their relevance or importance. Time is often wasted, and physicians are frustrated by computer-generated recommendations that don't make sense for particular patients.

Guidelines for Goal-Oriented Care

To be most useful for goal-oriented care, CPGs would be based upon goals and objectives rather than diseases. In their latest cardiovascular event prevention guideline, the American Heart Association and the American College of Cardiology took a step in that direction. They recommend that physicians and patients base decisions about statin therapy, not on cholesterol levels, but on risk of cardiovascular events. (Reducing the risk of cardiovascular events is an objective on the path toward prevention of premature death and disability).

That approach suggests that goal-oriented, outcomes-based guidelines are possible. The next small step forward would be a guideline summarizing what we know about how to prevent premature death and disability from cardiovascular events. Such a guideline should also provide tables and graphs showing the size of the benefits from various strategies by age, gender, and risk factor value (e.g., LDL and HDL cholesterol and blood pressure levels) and any other major mitigating or accentuating factors (e.g., smoking).

Quality of life improvement guidelines could summarize interventions proven to protect or improve various key functions like cognition, communication, and mobility. *The International Classification of Functioning, Disability, and Health* could serve as a useful guide. Reorienting guidelines in this way would not only be more helpful for person-centered decision-making, but it would reveal how little we know about how to help patients achieve meaningful goals, pointing out the need for additional research.

Goal-oriented care CPGs should also include evidence-based recommendations for how to analyze multiple risk factors, clarify and prioritize quality of life goals, support personal growth and development, and discuss, document, and disseminate advance directives.

Quality Measurement and Goal-Oriented Care

Goal-oriented care is most relevant to primary care. There is strong evidence that access to primary care — continuity, coordination, comprehensiveness, person-centeredness, integration, accountability — improves patient outcomes and reduces health costs. It therefore seems reasonable to measure the quality of primary care based upon those attributes.

When the care of patients is individualized, the quality of clinical decisions can only be fairly measured one patient at a time. That would obviously be more difficult than the current population-based method. However, assuming there are good reasons to measure quality, for example for continuous quality improvement within practices or health systems, there are some ways it could be done. Potential quality measures for evaluating goal-oriented care are listed in Table 8.1 (*see next page*). Obviously, the definitions, numerators, and denominators for each of these measures would have to be carefully defined.

One of the major objections physicians express about value-based reimbursement is that their ability to achieve the prescribed quality metrics is dependent upon their patients' willingness and ability to adhere to their recommendations. Goal-oriented care should be associated with improved adherence since care plans are co-created and linked to outcomes understood and valued by patients. When physicians and patients understand each other and collaborate effectively, patients are more likely to keep follow-up appointments and fill prescriptions on time. Adherence in this case would be to the individualized plans, not to population-based recommendations. Since better adherence is associated with better processes and outcomes of care, it might be an ideal measure of quality.

Table 8.1. Potential goal-oriented outcome measures

Measure (average across patient population)	Source/Calculation
Annual wellness visits	Claims data
Risk factor documentation (e.g., of risk factors in at least 5 categories)	Chart audit
Preventive services offered/provided	Claims data, chart audit, patient survey
High impact preventive services offered/provided	Claims data, chart audit, patient survey
Evidence of prioritization of preventive strategies based upon potential impact	Chart audit
Change in estimated life expectancy (ELE)	Poportionate hazards modeling using population statistics and data from RCTs of preventive strategies
Change in estimated health expectancy (EHE)	Method used to estimate ELE, adjusted for disability statistics
Documentation of living situation/conditions and any difficulties with essential functions	Chart audit, patient survey
Documentation of important, meaningful, and desired activities and relationships and any difficulties with participation	Chart audit, patient survey
Change in patient reported ability to participate in meaningful life activities	Patient survey
Change in patient self-rated health	Patient survey
Change in patient psychological resilience	Patient survey
Change in patient health literacy	Patient survey

Patient adherence to follow-up appointments, referral appointments, and prescription fills/refills	Chart audit, pharmacy records
Evidence of a discussion of end-of-life values and preferences	Chart audit, patient survey
Legal advance directives in primary care record	Chart audit, claims data
Quality of death	Family survey three-months after death

A Goal-Oriented Care Registry

Dr. Zsolt Nagykaldi at the University of Oklahoma has developed a goal-oriented registry focused primarily on prevention of premature death and disability. For each individual, the registry's computer program considers up to 215 different risk factors, then calculates current estimated life expectancy (ELE) and estimated health expectancy (EHE), a "real age," and a "wellness score." It then summarizes the patient's strengths and challenges and estimates the number of additional years of life the individual could gain by implementing all of the preventive measures recommended for them. Most importantly, it produces a list of preventive measures worth considering, showing the size of the expected benefit of each of them on additional life gained.

A typical report is shown below in Figure 8.1. Preliminary studies have found that people who receive the report and discuss it with their doctor receive more preventive services, more high impact preventive services, and increase their estimated life expectancy by approximately six months more over one year than those who complete the risk factor questionnaire but do not receive the report.

Figure 8.1: A Goal-Oriented Preventive
Services Registry Report

(45 years old - ELE: 81.1 - EHE: 74.6) ❓

Your estimated "**RealAge**" is: **45.3 years.**
This means that although your calendar age is
45 years, your body is as "old" in terms of risk,
as that of an average 45.3 year old in your
peer group (same age, gender, and ethnicity).

Your **Wellness Score is: 102.** A score of
90-100 means "average" health compared to
your peer group. Less than 90 shows worse
than average, while over 100 indicates better
than average health. The Score takes into
account both length and quality of life.

Your **Quality of Life & Health Score is:** *
Maximum score is 15 and the average is 12.

Your main health **strengths** are:
(assuming a fully completed HRA)

You had 16 or more years of education
You are employed
Your blood pressure is not significantly elevated
You eat a healthy and balanced diet
You are physically active
You do not smoke, drink too much, or abuse drugs
You have no family history of chronic conditions
You always buckle your seatbelt
You seem to be on top of your preventive services

Your main health **challenges** are:
(assuming a fully completed HRA)

Your life is stressful
You may need to address the amount of sleep you get
Your exposure to unhealthy materials is elevated
Your risk of injury from a car accident is elevated
You do not always wear a helmet when you should
Your risk of sexually transmitted disease may be elevated
**You may need to address the management of life
challenges**

Maximum **health benefit** that can be gained
when all services are completed or maintained:

6.91 additional years of life

Preventive services **ranked** in a decreasing
order of health benefit:

		Preventive Services	**Share of Benefit** ❓
Link to Resources	<--	Stress reduction	
Link to Resources	<--	Weight control	
Link to Resources	<--	Adjusting sleeping time	
Link to Resources	<--	Cholesterol measurement	
Link to Resources	<--	PAP smear	
Link to Resources	<--	Mammography	
Link to Resources	<--	Seatbelt use	
Link to Resources	<--	Sun exposure protection	
Link to Resources	<--	Adult dT-Tdap	
Link to Resources	<--	Folic acid supplementation	
Link to Resources	<--	Pneumonia vaccination	

*There is also a quality of life component, not shown here.

Chapter 9

Research

"I did then what I knew how to do. Now that I know better, I do better."

—Maya Angelou

"Your assumptions are your windows on the world. Scrub them off every once in a while, or the light won't come in."

—Isaac Asimov

OUR CONCEPTUAL FRAMEWORK INFLUENCES the questions we ask and the methods we use to answer them. Since medical research has primarily focused on questions related to problem-solving, research methods have been designed for that purpose, and that is what we know the most about. We know a lot about what can be done to correct abnormalities. We know less about what should be done to help people achieve their health goals, and because patient goals have received so little attention, we may know even less about how to elicit them and how to support the actions required to achieve them.

Prevention of Premature Death and Disability

Goal attainment differs from problem-solving in several ways. In the case of life extension, the timeline is obviously longer. The greatest challenge for researchers studying life extension is that health problems and risk factors often take years to cause death, and it has been hard for researchers to get funding to conduct studies lasting longer than three to five years. As a result, the actual benefits of many preventive measures can only be prospectively estimated from potentially life-limiting events like heart attacks.

Retrospective studies looking at exposure histories in people who have died are subject to a plethora of potential biases, not the least of which is the difficulty ascertaining the actual cause of death. Because autopsies are rarely performed anymore, the best available information on causes of death in the general population comes from death certificates, which, according to at least four studies conducted in the United States between 2005 and 2017, are often inaccurate. Supporting that view, a study conducted in 2012 in Norway found that an autopsy changed the cause of death in 61% of cases, and in 32% of cases, the change was considered major. A 2012 systematic review concluded that as many as 28% (40,500) adults who die in an intensive care unit in the United States each year are misdiagnosed.

Most of the information we have about the impact of health care on survival, therefore, pertains only to people with a single disease or set of risk factors that are likely to cause death within a short period of time. For most diseases, we don't really know whether treatment improves survival or by how much and at what cost.

Heaven help us when patients begin to ask reasonable questions like, "If I take this blood pressure medicine, and it lowers my blood pressure by 10mmHg, how much longer, on average, can I expect to stay alive free from serious disability? And how long will I need to take it to reap those benefits?" But, how can patients be expected to make truly informed decisions about life extension strategies, and how can physicians know when to suggest them, without that kind of information?

Implementation of a goal-oriented approach will require more information from a broader range of people followed over longer periods of time. This could be done prospectively or retrospectively. The accuracy of those studies would be enhanced by a renewed emphasis on autopsies, which increasingly can be done using advanced imaging techniques supplemented by needle biopsies rather than full body dissection. That information could enrich computer models like Archimedes (*https://www.healthaffairs.org/ doi/full/10.13777/hlthaff.2012.1063*), developed by Dr. David Eddy and colleagues, and predictive algorithms like the one developed by Dr. Nagykaldi.

Much of the information used in clinical care is limited by dichotomization of risk factors. Goal-oriented care will require information on risk and risk reduction across the full range of values for a given factor. We will need to know, for example whether risk reduction is the same across the full range of elevated blood pressures and the implication of diminishing returns. A common question that arises clinically is, "After reducing this patient's blood pressure from 200/110 to 150/95 with three antihypertensive medications, how much additional benefit can she expect to obtain by reducing it further?"

We need more information about trade-offs. In order to decide whether treatment of a disease is a good idea, a patient must not only consider whether the treatment could extend their life, but whether the life gained would be worth the effort. If sleeping an extra hour each night increased a patient's life expectancy by five months over a ten-year period, it would be important to know how much of that additional time would be spent asleep and whether there could be other beneficial effects that would make it worthwhile.

Current Quality of Life

It should now be clear that quality of life is defined very differently by different people. That creates at least two challenges for researchers. The first challenge is how to measure the success of a treatment intended to improve quality of life. The standard approach is to measure relief of symptoms, improvement in standard functions, physical signs, and test results — the same measures for every person enrolled in the study. However, there is no particular reason why the outcome of interest couldn't be different for each person as long as the measures of interest were defined prior to the experiment. For example, the outcome could be whether or not participants improved their ability to participate in the activities each considered important, like the man who wanted to go bow hunting.

The second challenge is that the strategies needed to improve quality of life are likely to be different for each individual. This challenge could be met by studying decision-making processes rather than specific strategies. For example, rather than studying whether a medicine or surgical procedure improves the abilities of participants to achieve their quality of life goals, researchers could study whether having an evaluation by an occupational therapist followed by an individualized treatment plan is more effective than the standard medical approach. By the way, when that kind of experiment has been done, occupational therapy has generally been shown to be more effective than standard care, which makes sense since improving quality of life is what occupational therapists are all about.

Personal Growth and Development

Personal growth and development have typically been studied by psychologists who have focused primarily on children. However, aside from the attention paid to developmental milestones during well-childcare visits and in mental health settings, that knowledge has had very little impact on health care. A goal-oriented approach would require better measures of personal growth and development at all ages and more studies examining the impact of interventions on them.

For example, health literacy is an area of personal growth and development defined as "the degree to which individuals have the capacity to obtain, process, and understand basic health information and services needed to make appropriate health decisions." Much has already been learned about how the health care system can both assess and improve health literacy, but more information is needed.

As mentioned in an earlier chapter, other health-related developmental areas needing further study include: 1) mastery of the skills required for healthy living; 2) increasing motivation to maintain and improve health; 3) strengthening the relational skills needed for integration within a social network; and 4) developing the habits of self-assessment, reflection, goal-setting, and self-directed learning.

Goal-oriented physicians and their patients would also benefit from knowing more about how to assess and enhance physiological and psychological resilience. A great deal of relevant information probably exists but, to my knowledge, it hasn't been analyzed from a goal-oriented perspective.

A Good Death

Though recommendations abound, surprisingly little research has been done to determine the best ways to improve the likelihood of experiencing a good death. As with quality of life, values and preferences for care at the end of life differ significantly, and so the outcomes of interest must be individualized. Since the end-of-life values of many people include impacts on family members, data should be routinely collected from them sometime after the death of a loved one. Again, studies should evaluate decision-making, documentation, and implementation processes in addition to standardized strategies like completion of formal advance directives.

Decision-Making Processes

To fully implement goal-oriented health care, physicians also need to know more about the process of goal-setting and strategic planning. Fortunately, other fields (e.g., education, mental health, financial planning, and business) have experience using a goal-oriented approach, and much of that knowledge should be applicable. However, some challenges would likely be unique to health care.

Section 3

Practicing Goal-Oriented Care

"Too often, educational curricula, instructional methods, and assessment techniques are so tightly constructed that learners have difficulty salvaging the human being – the doctor or the patient – from the educational package in which they are presented."

—Walker Percy, MD

IN THIS SECTION I WILL DISCUSS what goal-oriented care looks like in practice. Acknowledging the obstacles that exist within the health care system today, I will describe what I believe is currently possible, based largely upon my own clinical experience, while hinting at what could be possible in the future.

Chapter 10

Common Mistakes
and Misconceptions

*"Just as philosophy is the study of other people's misconceptions,
so history is the study of other people's mistakes."*
—Philip Guedalla

WHILE I HOPE THAT YOU NOW HAVE a general understanding of goal-oriented care, experience tells me that some of you may still have misconceptions. Before moving on to implementation, I want to address some common misconceptions and mistakes that physicians have expressed to me over the years.

Misconceptions

1. Some physicians have argued that goal-oriented care is simply a shift in semantics (i.e., exchanging the word *goals* for *problems*). Nothing could be further from the truth. Goals are fundamentally different from problems. Shifting the focus of attention from problem-solving to goal attainment changes the nature of both clinical decision-making and the physician-patient relationship. Problems can be detached from those who are experiencing them. It is entirely reasonable to hold a conference on Parkinson's Disease without ever mentioning a specific patient. Goals, on the other hand, can't be separated from those who aspire to them. It would be hard to discuss a goal-oriented plan for a

patient with Parkinson's Disease without knowing about that person.

When taken out of the context of goal achievement, risk reduction could be equated to problem-solving. Within a goal-oriented conceptual framework, however, they are viewed differently. While problem-solving is restorative, risk reduction is aspirational, and while problem-solving is often viewed as an end in itself, risk reduction is a means to an end. Because risk reduction is directly connected to a desired outcome, all risk factors must be considered collectively, and that makes prioritization possible.

As discussed in previous chapters, full implementation of goal-oriented care principles will require substantial changes in record keeping, coding and billing, guidelines, quality metrics, and research methodologies. Significant gaps in our knowledge base will need to be filled. The very fact that those statements are true is evidence that this is not simply a change in semantics.

2. When attempting to incorporate goal setting into clinical care, some physicians, particularly geriatricians, often focus almost entirely on quality of life goals. Their arguments are that 1) quality of life is more important in old age than survival, and 2) life-prolonging strategies aren't very effective in the elderly anyway. While there is some validity to those arguments, it seems to me that ignoring the other three goals (preventing premature death/disability; maximizing personal growth and development; improving the chances of having a good death) and the trade-offs involved is short-sighted and unlikely to be acceptable to many older patients or their physicians.

3. A related misconception is that goal-oriented care only, or mostly, applies to the care of the elderly and other complex or "multi-problem" patients. I will acknowledge that the benefits of goal-oriented care may be greatest for those patients. However, as a way of thinking, it can be applied to anyone. Arguments in favor of beginning goal-oriented thinking at birth include: the much greater benefits that can be obtained from engaging in healthy behaviors as early in life as pos-

sible; the cumulative effect of successful growth and development strategies; and the importance, as stated earlier, of establishing advance directives prior to a catastrophic event.

4.   Another misconception is that goal-oriented care means finding out what patients identify as their goals and trying to help them achieve them. Goals are powerful because they provide direction. They also create alignment between physician and patient. For those positive things to happen, goals must be formulated from information provided by both, or in the case of a team or engaged family, all parties. They must account for the values, preferences, resources, and limitations of the patient as well as the medical knowledge, experience, and wisdom of the physician or team. As stated in an earlier chapter, patients are inclined to overvalue quality of life, so physicians must counterbalance that bias by emphasizing prevention. In the end, all involved must agree and commit to working toward the same goals.

Dr. David Waters, a psychologist who taught goal-oriented care principles to residents at the University of Virginia in the 1980s and 1990s, used the following example. Consider that you own a trekking company. Customers pay to take guided trips to the top of a mountain. They can choose between an easy path, a moderately strenuous one, or one that requires serious mountain climbing expertise. Since you will be their guide on the trek, you explain the choices, ask for their opinion, and then try to determine how much help they are likely to need. You won't agree to take someone who requires a cane on the moderately strenuous hike, and you won't take someone with no climbing experience on the steepest trail. Similarly, as a goal-oriented physician, you should generally not agree to support a plan that has little chance of succeeding, especially if it could be dangerous. A corollary is that if you find you are working harder than the patient, you need to back up and recalibrate.

5. Once a physician has concluded that goal-oriented care offers important advantages over their current approach, the first reason given

for not implementing it is that it would require too much time. Some visits will certainly be longer. For example, preventive care will require at least one long visit per year, but many physicians and Medicare already recommend an annual wellness visit. Goal-oriented care places greater responsibility on patients, including homework assignments (e.g., surveys, advance directives, etc.), potentially reducing physician time. Visits focused on quality of life goals need not be longer than thoughtful problem-oriented visits. None of the examples I have provided throughout the book required more time, simply a different mindset and different questions. However, as with any other skill set, maximal efficiency requires training and experience. There will, of course be patients who need a great deal more time than others. In those cases, a problem-oriented approach might save time at the expense of effective person-centered care. Much of the additional work required in such cases could be done by non-physicians.

6. Some physicians who hear or read about goal-oriented care worry that, if they adopt this approach, they might miss something clinically important. Although extra caution is warranted when implementing such a major change in approach, there is no reason why goal-oriented care, once mastered, should be less scientifically rigorous. It simply provides a different framework within which to fit clinically relevant information. In fact, the Problem List doesn't go away entirely. It is incorporated into a compendium of risk factors for premature death and disability and obstacles relevant to current quality of life and personal growth and development. However, it is no longer used to organize most visits.

7. The final misconception is that most good primary care clinicians already provide goal-oriented care. My experience and some preliminary research conducted by Dr. Becky Purkaple tells me that is not generally true. However, I do believe that physicians who have cared for the same patients over long periods of time begin to think in terms of patient goals because they become increasingly invested in the outcomes. Some have

told me they had to discard much of what they learned in medical school and residency in order to develop a different way of thinking and behaving, but they can't describe exactly what they do differently. For those physicians who have already figured out how to provide goal-oriented care, I hope this book will provide the language and concepts they have been looking for so that they can teach others to do it.

Mistakes

1. Because of misconceptions about goal-oriented care, there are several mistakes that physicians tend to make when trying to implement it. The most common mistake is to attach goals to problems or to groups of patients defined by the number of problems they have. For example, a physician might say, "The goals for this patient's diabetes are ..." Goal-oriented care does not begin with a problem. It begins with goals. Problems are viewed as obstacles or challenges that must be faced to achieve those goals. A typical care plan looks like this:

Problems	Goals	Strategies	Person Responsible
Type 2 Diabetes	Prevent micro-vascular damage/ events	Keep A1c below 7.5%	Physician and patient

A goal-oriented care plan for the same patient might look like this:

Goals	Obstacles	Strategies	Person Responsible
Increase ability to play with grandchildren	Mild dehydra-tion due to hyperglycemia	Keep blood sugar levels below 200mg/dl	Physician and patient
Reduce risk of future disability	Hyperglycemia as a risk factor for microvascu-lar complications	Keep A1c below 7.5%	Physician and patient

In the above example, the difference may not appear to be significant, but it is. The first care plan is physician-centered, the second person-centered.

2. A second mistake that physicians make involves confusing strategies and objectives with goals. A goal is a desired outcome that can stand alone without qualifications. That is, it makes no sense to ask, "Why would you want that to happen?" An objective is a measurable step on the path toward a goal. A strategy is an action taken to achieve an objective. Lowering blood pressure is a strategy for reducing the risk of strokes, kidney and heart failure, and heart attacks. Lowering the risk of those adverse events are objectives, and prevention of premature death and disability are the goals. That distinction is critical because it is goals that encourage creative care planning, goals that create patient-physician collaboration, and goals that drive behavior change.

3. Because physicians are so used to creating problem lists, it is only natural that some would assume that goal-oriented care involves creating a goals list, and that establishing goals is like making diagnoses. There is no need for a goals list. There are only four major goals. They need to be personalized and prioritized, and that information should be recorded in the record, but it doesn't make sense to put them on a list. Because the strategies required for each of the goals are different, it could make sense to divide the record into four parts, one for each goal area.

4. It is important to understand that goal achievement is probably not as important as the process of working toward goals collaboratively. It doesn't make sense to spend an inordinate amount of time trying to get the goals and strategies right from the outset. More important than initial goal-setting are the adjustments made subsequently as lessons are learned during implementation.

Legitimate Concerns

In addition to the obstacles mentioned in the prior section, there are some legitimate reasons physicians should be concerned about adopting goal-oriented care. It isn't cookbook medicine. It requires more creative energy and a somewhat greater fund of knowledge, akin to the difference between solving a math problem and using math to build a better squirrel trap. Determining whether an abnormality can be corrected is insufficient; there is also the question of whether it should be corrected.

Returning to the example of acute upper respiratory infections, the question of whether the causative agent is viral or bacterial is largely irrelevant since the vast majority of these infections are self-limited. The more important concern is whether it is safe, perhaps safer, to delay treatment in order to avoid adverse effects and allow the patient's immune system to have a chance to react and become stronger.

Goal-oriented care also requires greater interpersonal skills and a more significant emotional investment. Depending upon the personality of the physician, this could be emotionally enriching or exhausting. However, the physician burnout rate is rising, and most concur that it has something to do with our current approach to care. While a cookie-cutter approach may conserve energy, it isn't necessarily cognitively, psychologically, or professionally rewarding.

Goal-Oriented Care as a Conceptual Framework

Several other approaches to person-centered care have been proposed including narrative medicine and relationship-based care. In addition, novel approaches to problem-oriented care, such as functional medicine, complementary and alternative medicine, and personalized medicine based upon genomics, are being articulated based upon advances in our understanding of human biology. These methods can be all be applied, if helpful, within the conceptual framework of goal-oriented care.

Chapter 11

Primary Care
and Primary Health Care

"Our primary health care should begin on the farm and in our hearts, not in some laboratory of the biotech and pharmaceutical companies."

—Gary Hopkins

"The mission of primary care is to help each person experience a full, meaningful, and rewarding life."

—Barbara Starfield

Primary Care

WHILE GOAL-ORIENTED CARE IS APPLICABLE to all health care professionals, it is most relevant to those who care for patients over long periods of time. That includes primary care clinicians and clinicians who take care of patients with long-term special needs (e.g., patients with HIV, certain genetic abnormalities, some cancers, and end-stage renal failure). It is in those settings, where relationships are most important, when goals and care plans are most helpful.

Though not necessarily more time-consuming than problem-solving, goal-setting and care planning are complex tasks. The health professional or professionals involved must have a broad understanding of clinical medicine and the health care system in order to provide appropriate guidance. They must also be in a position to influence the actions of other professionals within the system (e.g., referral special-ists, hospitalists, rehabilitation therapists, and counselors). Therefore, it is vital, in my opinion, that physicians be involved. The roles re-quired of primary care physicians in a goal-oriented health care system will be more important, more challenging, and more rewarding. The job will require our brightest, best-trained, and most empathic individ-uals, people who are able to help their patients integrate large amounts of information to make well-reasoned decisions that are both feasible and in their best interest.

Once a plan is set in motion, particularly if the strategies are mul-tiple or difficult, care coordination becomes critical. Depending upon the patient and their plan, care coordination may require the skills of a nurse or a social worker. Of course, if the tasks are primarily admin-istrative in nature, coordination can be handled by office staff.

Physician extenders are invaluable in primary care. They are able to fill a number of critical roles that increase access, coordination, con-tinuity, and comprehensiveness of care. Because nurse practitioners have been through nursing school, they have a somewhat different and complementary set of knowledge, skills, and attitudes than physicians. Within a physician-led team, nurse practitioners and physician assis-tants can serve a valuable role in both acute and chronic care manage-ment.

Two other types of health care professionals could be invaluable to a goal-oriented primary care team. Because the health challenges that people face often involve mood, anxiety, and sleep disorders, unhealthy behaviors, and troubling relationships, mental health professionals can be particularly helpful, especially if they are skilled in cognitive behav-ioral therapy and behavior modification techniques.

Though rarely included in primary care practices in the U.S., occupa-tional and physical therapists could provide the additional knowledge and skills needed to expand the capacity of the team to help patients achieve quality of life goals. They could be particularly helpful to older patients and children with developmental disabilities. Occupational therapists, in particular, are already trained to provide goal-oriented care. In their absence on the primary care team, it is essential that primary care physicians know what they have to offer and establish close referral relationships with them.

Primary Health Care

In 1978, the World Health Organization (WHO), following its meeting in Kazakhstan, produced a groundbreaking document called the Alma-Ata Declaration. In it, the WHO defined a new term, *primary health care*, as "essential health care based on practical, scientifically sound and socially acceptable methods and technology made universally available to individuals and families in the community through their full participation and at a cost that the community and country can afford to maintain at every stage of their development in the spirit of self-reliance and self-determination." The Declaration states that "primary health care involves, in addition to the health sector, all related sectors and aspects of national and community development, in particular agriculture, animal husbandry, food, industry, education, housing, public works, communications and other sectors; and demands the coordinated efforts of all those sectors."

Based upon that conceptualization, primary care represents only one component of primary health care. Unfortunately, in the United States at least, coordination and alignment of the key primary health care sectors in most communities is inadequate. During my final 15 years as an academician, much of my time was spent trying to help primary care practices improve their processes of care. In one project, my team and I focused on improving the number and quality of well-child visits. In one county, many low-income children were being immunized at the county health department and never getting a full well-child visit. The primary care practices were upset because they were being penalized by the Medicaid program for not doing the recommended number of well-child visits. They also believed that the children weren't getting optimal care.

The medical director of the county health department was concerned that children weren't going to get their immunizations if the health department nurses didn't administer them when the mothers and children were there for the Special Supplemental Nutrition Program for Women, Infants, and Children (WIC) visits. He claimed that parents had complained that it was hard to get appointments with their primary care doctors. He also believed the health department was better qualified to give immunizations than most primary care practices. He said they always recommended to parents that their children should also be seen for well-child visits. When I suggested that the community physicians might be willing to see their Medicaid patients at the health department, he said that wouldn't be possible because it would involve mixing public and private funds.

There are also significant barriers to collaboration between primary care practices and mental health professionals, though major efforts are now being made to address them. In another project, we tried to improve the recognition and treatment of primary care patients with depression. The evidence suggested the need for a care coordinator who would make sure depressed patients filled their prescriptions and/or kept their counseling appointments and were improving. The county probably only needed one full-time person to fill that position, shared among the six primary care practices and the community mental health center. We identified a source of funding for such a person, but the community couldn't figure out who the care coordinator's employer should be.

The Centers for Disease Control and Prevention has encouraged state departments of health to develop health improvement plans. In some states, county health improvement plans (CHIPs) are consolidated into the state health improvement plan (SHIP). Data from a variety of sources including community surveys are used to create these plans. However, the primary care sector is rarely involved and often not even aware of this activity. Planning meetings are typically held during the workday when physicians are seeing patients. Data from primary care practices is typically not available to public health staff. Not-for-profit hospitals that accept Medicare or Medicaid are also required to conduct community needs assessments periodically. Again, primary care practices are generally not involved.

A goal-oriented approach could be used as a framework for integration across primary health care sectors. Working together effectively across traditional disciplinary and organizational boundaries requires agreement on and commitment to common goals. The goals I have proposed for individuals probably apply equally well to communities. Effective strategies would, of course, include community-based interventions. Algorithms based upon community strengths, risk factors, and priorities could be created to guide decision making.

When I have informed primary care physicians about the assessment and planning going on in their communities, they almost always ask, "Why wasn't I invited to participate?" When I have posed that question to those in charge of the assessment and planning process, they either tell me that the physicians had been invited and declined or that they agreed but didn't participate. If you want to become involved, the best first contact point is likely to be the medical director of the county health department. Explain your schedule and availability for meetings and ask if there are ways to stay involved even if you can't always attend the meetings. Your input and data should be extremely valuable to the process.

Consultations and Referrals

When a patient has a sustained relationship with a competent goal-oriented primary care physician, other health care professionals can, for the most part, continue to provide problem-oriented care as long as there is good communication. However, goal-oriented care requires greater precision when communicating patient goals and the limits of consultation and referral requests. For example, "Mr. Ellerbe and I are hopeful that you can confirm the cause of his shoulder pain, which we think is a partial tear of his supraspinatus tendon, and suggest non-operative ways he can treat it so that he can continue to play basketball. If an operation is a reasonable option, please advise him about the recovery time and probability that he can return to basketball."

An important responsibility of primary care physicians is to serve as a patient advocate. Mary's story provides a good example.

Mary had undergone two coronary artery bypass procedures to relieve angina, the most recent one seven years ago. Her angina had returned and was again unrelieved by medications. It prevented her from performing even simple tasks. I referred her back to the cardiac surgeon who had performed the prior procedures, but he told her he wouldn't operate again because her risk of death during surgery was greater than 20%. She subsequently told me she was willing to take that risk since her life was no longer worth living, given the severity of her symptom. After discussing the situation with her surgeon, he wouldn't change his mind, so I referred her to another surgeon who operated. Fortunately, Mary survived the operation, and her angina and ability to care for herself improved.

Within a goal-oriented health care system, subspecialists and other consultants would have somewhat less freedom to act independently. They would need to trust the primary care process that resulted in the consultation or referral and respect the requests made in the referral note. Deviations from requested services would need to be discussed with and approved by the referring physician and patient as in the following example.

Alvin had undergone coronary artery bypass surgery three years earlier for coronary artery disease. His cardiac surgeon requested that he come in for annual follow-up visits during which he would undergo cardiac stress testing. Since he was asymptomatic, I couldn't understand why it would matter if his stress test was positive, since the only significant benefit of opening up obstructed coronary arteries is symptom reduction. I called the surgeon, who acknowledged that the stress testing was probably unnecessary, though he thought the evidence of benefit for patients like Alvin might be incomplete. After we discussed the options, Alvin decided not to have the test since there was some cost and risk involved. He said he would rather not know if his obstruction was getting worse, since he was already doing what he could to prevent heart attacks. Had Alvin's surgeon insisted on doing the test, Alvin and I would have discussed whether he should find a different surgeon and, in fact, whether annual visits to a cardiac surgeon were even necessary.

Patient Responsibilities

Within a goal-oriented health care system, patients will have additional responsibilities as well. They will need to establish a longitudinal relationship with a primary care physician they trust and show up for annual wellness visits, having completed their homework assignment and having thought about and discussed their values and preferences with family or significant others.

In my geriatric continuity clinic, patients were required to complete a 24-page questionnaire before enrollment and a 14-page update each year prior to their wellness visit. The average age of the patients seen in that clinic was 78. Many of them had cognitive impairment and required assistance from family members or, occasionally, our nurses. Only one patient that I am aware of refused to complete the initial questionnaire. The reason she gave was that she didn't want me to know that much about her.

Patients will be encouraged to learn as much as possible about their health challenges and vulnerabilities, join relevant national and local associations, join online discussion groups, and bring new information to their physicians. A rehabilitation physician once told me, "You have to *learn* to live with a chronic illness." Patients will therefore be expected to be prepared to engage in discussions about their goals and what they would be willing to do to achieve them.

In order to measure progress, patients will need to maintain diaries and learn to monitor key physiological parameters. When considering long-term medications for management of symptoms, they will need to be willing to participate in simple N-of-1 trials to document the size of the benefits they receive from them. When they are seen by other health care professionals, they will be responsible for informing their primary care physician, and they will be expected to discuss new recommendations with their primary care physician. The following is an example of how that can work.

George was referred by his primary care physician to a proctologist for surgical resection of an anal fistula. As part of the evaluation, the proctologist recommended a barium enema to rule out Crohn's Disease, which can cause anal fistulas and impair healing following resection. Before agreeing to have the X-rays, George called his primary care physician. He reported he had had absolutely no symptoms of Crohn's Disease and was willing to take the small risk of impaired healing to avoid the discomfort and cost of a barium enema. His primary care physician advised him to refuse the test and have the proctologist call him if that was a problem. The proctologist was agreeable, and the procedure went well.

Conflicting Values

The process of goal-setting is collaborative. Physician and patient are in it together. Both are invested in making the plan work. That means there will sometimes be conflicts. Of course, conflicts occur in problem-oriented care also, but they are less likely to be recognized.

Edith was a 66-year-old widow who I took care of long before I began to think about goal-oriented care. She had type 2 diabetes mellitus, with blood sugar levels consistently between 225 and 300 despite all of my dietary and pharmacological interventions. She came in weekly to turn in her home blood sugar readings and have her blood pressure and fingerstick blood sugar checked by one of our nurses. (This was before hemoglobin A1c testing). She saw me once a month to review her results and make medication adjustments.

Because her blood sugar results never improved despite my best efforts, I decided to hospitalize her. (It was before current restrictions on hospitalizations). In the hospital, her blood sugars were completely normal on the very same diet I had advised and the medicines she was supposed to be taking at home. When I pointed that out to her and told her as respectfully as I could that all she needed to do was follow my previous advice and her diabetes would be under control, she fired me. It was only later, in conversations with my nurse, that I found out Edith had been intentionally keeping her blood sugars above 200 so she would have a reason to come to the office every week. It was a major social event in her otherwise lonely life. Had I known, I might have been able to justify weekly visits for her despite normal blood sugars.

An issue about which my patients and I often disagreed was cigarette smoking. When patients chose to continue to smoke, expressing awareness that they were sacrificing months or even years of life, I agreed to continue being their physician if they agreed to allow me to bring up smoking cessation periodically. They nearly always agreed. Some subsequently stopped smoking, and others didn't.

Chapter 12

Goal-Oriented Care Processes*

Annual Wellness Visits

GOAL-ORIENTED CARE IS FUTURE-ORIENTED. Physicians must always consider the long-term effects of their recommendations. Helping a patient with an acute upper respiratory tract infection, for example, should include education about how to reduce the risk of future infections and what to do about them when they happen.

Prevention and end-of-life goals involve outcomes far in the future, so decision-making can be scheduled. I found it particularly helpful to schedule periodic visits focused entirely on prevention of premature death and disability and end-of-life planning. Fortunately, Medicare and many other health insurance companies have now agreed to pay for such visits, though they sometimes limit payment to primary and secondary prevention, requiring creative coding and billing strategies. Patients with few codable health challenges can be billed for a wellness visit, while those with multiple codable challenges can be charged for a comprehensive medical visit. For very complex patients, it sometimes makes sense to schedule both a wellness visit and a separate comprehensive medical visit.

---

*NOTE: *This chapter is intended mainly for primary care physicians and the other members of primary care teams.*

While several published meta-analyses have found that annual wellness visits are of no value, studies that only included wellness visits done in primary care settings in which some form of prioritization (e.g., health risk appraisal) and behavioral counseling were included have documented increased implementation of key preventive services and increased average estimated or actual life expectancies.

Because these visits typically take between 30 and 60 minutes, it is important to calculate the number you can do and still be able to see patients for acute illnesses and quality of life visits. That calculation requires an estimate of total panel size and the age distribution of your panel. A physician with 2,000 active patients, half of whom are over the age of fifty, might estimate that annual visits for older patients would take 1,000 hours per year and those with younger patients an additional 500 hours. Since there are approximately 2,000 hours per year available for patient care, decisions might have to be made about reducing panel size, starting wellness visits at the age of 21 rather than at 2, or making some visits more efficient/shorter by having others in the office do parts or all of them.

It is also important to decide how best to distribute such visits across the year and across each day. In a typical practice, it makes sense to schedule them once a year during the month of each patient's birth. In a university or vacation town it might make sense to do more of them during times when acute visit rates are lower (i.e., when school is out, or the weather is poor). Because these visits take longer than acute care visits, no-shows are a bigger problem. Reminder calls are almost essential. Some physicians charge for the visit unless the patient cancels at least 24 hours in advance. Others fill the space with walk-ins and work-ins.

I found it important to have patients do homework in preparation for their annual wellness visits. At a minimum, patients should be asked to review and update their risk factors and the preventive measures taken to reduce them. More complex patients, or perhaps patients over 50, should also review and update their past medical and surgical histories.

At the visit, all risk factors for premature death are reviewed, from social and environmental determinants, to behavioral risk factors, to biological and psychological requirements, to risk factors for cancer and cardiovascular events, to current medical challenges. A prioritized preventive plan is then constructed based upon the potential impact of available risk reduction strategies and patient preferences and abilities.

All adults should also be asked to respond to several questions about end-of-life values and preferences. I found reviewing their written answers to be a comfortable way to initiate further conversation about advance directives. The two most important pieces of information for planning end-of-life care are: 1) conditions viewed by the patient as worse than death, and 2) the name of a surrogate decision-maker who understands the patient's values and preferences. However, when asked, most patients have a number of other issues they would like to discuss.

Because end-of-life values and preferences are often complex and sensitive, patients should be asked to think about and discuss them at home with family members prior to and between annual wellness visits. Suggestions about how to initiate those conversations can be found at http://www.dyingmatters.org/page/resources-talking-about-death-and-dying, at www.fivewishes.org, and on the PREPARE website at https://prepareforyourcare.org. There is also a wonderful game families or friends can play called "Hello" (www.commonpractice.com), developed at the Penn State Hershey Medical Center, which can help patients and future surrogate decision-makers discover their values and preferences about end-of-life care.

A variety of non-legal documents have also been created to help patients think about their values and preferences. One example is the Values History originally developed at the University of New Mexico, which can be found at https://cdn.ymaws.com/www.hospicefed.org/resource/resmgr/hpcfm_pdf_doc/valueshistoryform.pdf, but you can easily create your own form to collect the kinds of information you have found to be most helpful. A useful HIPPA compliance site for documenting and sharing values, preferences, and directives with health care providers is located at www.mydirectives.com.

Wellness visits for children include a variety of important tasks. It is important to emphasize those likely to have the greatest impact. In full term infants, a major focus should be on family relationships and parenting skills since development of trust is so incredibly important to future quality of life and possibly life expectancy. The "typical day" question is a good way to begin that conversation.

The two most frequent causes of death in young children in the United States are motor vehicle accidents and gunshot wounds; third is cancer, followed by suffocation, drowning, and poisoning. For that reason, safety issues should be emphasized to parents, and justified based upon the physician's responsibility to try to prevent premature death and disability. It is also a good time to encourage physical activity and healthy eating and sleeping behaviors.

Adolescents are risk-takers. The leading causes of death in teenagers are accidents, homicides, and suicides. Taking reasonable risks is important for psychological development, and it is important that teens make mistakes and experience failure. Success in life depends upon being able to overcome obstacles and learn from mistakes. While most mistakes can be corrected or overcome, a few can't. Becoming addicted to drugs, nicotine, or alcohol; being involved in a preventable car accident or shooting in which someone is injured or killed; developing an incurable sexually transmitted disease; and having or causing an unwanted pregnancy are examples of mistakes that can have long-term negative effects on a person's life.

Once again, preventive care conversations with teens and their parents can begin with a statement like, "I assume you are here because you want me to help [child's name] stay alive and healthy." Assuming agreement, it is usually helpful then to ask parents to step outside and ask the adolescent about hopes, dreams, and plans, and then about risk-taking, making mistakes, and overcoming obstacles. All adolescents should be routinely screened for symptoms of depression, sexual activity, and use of addictive substances. Having teens complete a pre-visit questionnaire on a computer tablet can sometimes facilitate discussion.

With parent(s) present, it makes sense to discuss those factors that can support autonomy while reducing the chance that the adolescent's risk-taking will result in avoidable tragedy. Those include encouragement to become involved in safe activities; keeping close track of where they are and who they are with; having reasonable rules with consequences; emphasizing positive values; staying connected and providing opportunities for conversation; and helping them rehearse saying no to unwanted and potentially dangerous invitations. They also include parental gun safety measures and awareness of online activities.

Quality of Life

As in problem-oriented care, most patient encounters will involve challenges to patients' quality of life. When a problem-solving strategy is what is needed, goal-oriented care and problem-oriented care will look similar. In goal-oriented care, however, even acute problems are considered within the context of the patient's life course and are viewed as obstacles or challenges to be faced, providing opportunities to address personal growth and development.

Sam was 67 years old when he suffered his first stroke. When I met him on the inpatient rehabilitation center where I was attending, he had a right hemiplegia and was despondent. After establishing rapport, we talked about his life prior to the stroke and challenges he had faced in the past. He was a Vietnam veteran and had overcome several major financial challenges to ultimately have a good marriage, help raise two happy and successful children, and be able to retire at age 66. Together we were able to reframe the stroke as another major challenge in his life, which he then approached with a sense of optimism based upon his record of having successfully overcome major challenges in the past.

While attending on that same rehabilitation unit, another faculty physician asked me, "Don't you get tired of strokes and amputations?" The question took me aback. I had never thought about it that way. For me, every patient was unique. Their diagnoses didn't define them. I viewed their current difficulties within the context of their life stories, each of which was unique, interesting, and relevant.

Symptom Diaries and N-of-1 Trials

When asked, patients often aren't sure whether a medicine they have been taking for years is helping them. Because of the placebo effect and the hazards of therapies, particularly medicines, it is essential to know whether they are beneficial. There are two ways to find out. The first is to have the patient keep a diary for several weeks prior to and several weeks following initiation of any new, long-term medicine as a practice policy. The diary should include the symptoms of concern, ability to perform desired activities, most likely adverse effects of the therapy, and a few unrelated adverse symptoms or events. While that doesn't eliminate the possibility of the placebo effect, it creates a permanent record of the perceived benefits and short-term hazards of the strategy for later review when deciding to try changing or abandoning the strategy. The same diary can be used across time to evaluate the continued need for the medicine.

An even better approach, though more difficult, is to conduct N-of-1 trials in which patients are given a medicine and a similar-looking placebo to take on alternate days or weeks, depending upon the stability of the symptom and half-life of the medicine, until they determine which works better for them. Obviously, this usually requires the help of a pharmacist.

Care Pathways

Goal-oriented care inspires greater investment on the parts of both patients and their physicians. Physician advice is rarely sufficient for goal achievement. Strategies must be carefully thought through and adjusted as necessary. Each plan of care will be unique, but there will be commonalities as well. For frequently occurring strategies, such as smoking cessation, blood pressure reduction, or blood glucose control, it can be helpful to develop standard clinical care pathways.

Some care pathways can be initiated and managed within the practice by an individual or team appropriate to the pathway. In those cases, printed algorithms or computer templates and standing orders are useful. Other pathways will need to be coordinated with outside individuals or organizations, requiring carefully written instructions.

One way to organize your thoughts as you design these pathways is to consider the eight attributes of primary care: accessibility, coordination, sustained care, comprehensiveness, partnership with patients, person-centeredness, integration, and accountability. For example:

Accessibility: Pathways should be accessible to any patient who might benefit. The entry point need not be a wellness visit. When possible, accommodations should be included for patients with access barriers including language barriers, reduced health literacy, transportation problems, and disabilities.

Coordination: There must be a process for communication among those involved both inside and outside the practice so that everyone can track the patient's progress along the pathway.

Sustained Care: Each pathway should have a designated coordinator. Depending upon staffing, that could be the physician, a mid-level clinician, a nurse, a social worker, a mental health professional, a medical assistant, or a non-clinical staff person. Alerts should be built into the pathways that notify the physician when a patient is having difficulty.

Comprehensiveness: Checklists should be included to make sure that all options are considered.

Partnership with Patients: It should be clear that the practice is invested in patients' successes including agreements to monitor progress, answer questions, and detect adverse effects. Periodic phone calls to the patient to check on their progress have been found to be a very effective strategy for detecting obstacles early when they can be circumvented.

Person-centeredness: The pathways must be adaptable to personal habits, preferences, resources, and limitations. It should be easy for the physician to make individual modifications when indicated.

Integration: A component of the pathways should be a checklist of potential hazards and interactions with other health challenges, risk factors, and medications.

Accountability: Clinicians and staff involved in a pathway should receive training and maintain competence in the functions assigned to them. Patients' successes and failures should be tracked over time and periodic modifications made to the pathways to align with newer evidence and to maximize positive outcomes.

I recognize that well-organized clinical pathways are not the norm currently, at least not in outpatient settings. This book is about a new way of thinking, which leads to new ways of organizing what we do. Constructing clinical pathways is very possible in many settings without major changes in staffing or funding. To some degree, the use of clinical pathways depends upon the concept of prioritization, which is a central feature of goal-oriented care.

Teamwork

Health care has evolved to a point of complexity where teamwork has become essential. Of course, teamwork has always been important in certain areas like intensive care, the operating room, and rehabilitation settings, but it is now becoming a central feature of newer models of primary care and within integrated health systems. Aside from organizational and training requirements, the most important prerequisite for effective teamwork is agreement on a common set of patient-relevant goals. In primary care, patients are essential team members.

As a practical matter, it isn't always possible or even desirable for all members of a health care team to meet in the same place at the same time. One of the most important organizational challenges raised by goal-oriented care is construction of methods to facilitate asynchronous interdisciplinary teamwork. Whenever possible, that should involve direct person-to-person interactions among team members (e.g., huddles) to supplement medical record notes. However, full team meetings with patient and sometimes family involvement will sometimes be necessary.

On our inpatient geriatric rehabilitation unit, I participated regularly in interdisciplinary care planning meetings. The ostensible purpose of those meetings was to establish patient goals. However, neither patients nor their family members were ever in attendance. The case manager typically went around the table asking the representative of each discipline – nursing, social work, physical therapy, occupational therapy, speech therapy, and medicine – in turn to state their goals for the patient. There was rarely any cross-disciplinary discussion. Each discipline had its area of expertise, and the boundaries between them were clearly defined by professional accreditation guidelines and local precedent. Though all members of the team sat at the same table at the same time, they were not a team. A problem-solving orientation tends to favor that sort of fragmented care.

By contrast, goal-oriented care directs everyone's efforts toward patients' goals, which cannot be owned by any one health care discipline. Elucidation of goals and priorities and the strategic planning that follows, more closely resembles brainstorming than traditional shared decision-making. Generally, more than one discipline is able to contribute to the discussion, and, of course, the patient is the final decision-maker.

Adjustments

All initial care plans are experimental. Strategies that seemed reasonable turn out to be impossible to carry out, objectives that seemed motivational lose their appeal, and even goals sometimes need to be reconsidered. In addition, patients' circumstances change. Adjustments are almost always required. It is therefore important, whenever a plan is developed, to negotiate a time interval after which it will be reassessed. These visits should generally be with the health care professional who helped the patient develop the plan.

Lists

Until a goal-oriented record is developed, it will be hard to avoid completing a Problem List. In goal-oriented care, the Problem List is best viewed as a list of risk factors, vulnerabilities, and potential obstacles and challenges to quality of life and a good death. With the exception of annual wellness visits, I used it as a memory jogger primarily, not as a way to organize patient encounters. The Medication List is obviously still important and should include both prescription and non-prescription medicines and supplements.

There is no need to create a Goals List. The same four goals apply to all patients until the prevention goal drops out. Objectives and strategies are embedded in the encounter and care planning notes and shouldn't require a designated list. Clinical care pathways will often include checklists to make sure all contraindications and options are considered.

Chapter 13

Changing the Conversation

"To speak a language is to take on a world, a culture."
—Frantz Fanon

"Never underestimate the power of words to heal and reconcile relationships."
—H. Jackson Brown

CHANGING PARADIGMS REQUIRES changing the language that we use. The following are some of the words that shape the current problem-oriented medical paradigm.

Words Used in Problem-Oriented Care but not in Goal-Oriented Care*

Normal: Falling within a variable middle range, depending upon the type of measurement or observation (e.g., for laboratory tests this is approximately 1 standard deviation on either side of the mean) of what is typically seen in a healthy (non-diseased) subset of the general population.

Problem: An abnormality of biochemistry, physiology, anatomy, or be-

---

NOTE: These definitions are my own, based upon common clinical usage. They may or may not correspond precisely to those found in dictionaries.

havior that results or could result in undesirable symptoms, signs, or other adverse outcomes.

Disease: A cluster of abnormal symptoms or signs that have a known or presumed common cause (e.g., Sickle Cell Disease, rheumatoid arthritis).

Syndrome: A set of two or more symptoms of unknown cause or causes that occur together in a sufficient number of people and cause enough discomfort to warrant a label (e.g., restless legs syndrome, dry eyes syndrome).

Morbidity: The non-fatal adverse physical and psychological consequences of a disease or syndrome.

Multi-morbidity: The adverse consequences, generally on an individual, of more than one disease or syndrome.

Treatment: A proposed solution to a health problem.

Management: Treatments that may alleviate symptoms and bring signs and test results closer to normal but will probably not result in a permanent solution to the problem.

Compliance: The degree to which a patient follows the recommendations of the health care team.

Adherence: A slightly less critical-sounding word for *compliance*.

Palliative care: Care, generally at or near the end of life, which focuses primarily on quality of life—especially comfort—for the patient and caregivers and on preparation for a comfortable death.

Words Used in Goal-Oriented Care

Goal: A desired outcome that can stand on its own merits. That is, it makes little sense to ask, "Why would you want that to happen?" The word *goal* is rarely used in conversations with patients. It is simply a way to describe the concepts involved in goal-oriented care.

Objective: A measurable and/or documentable step along the path toward a goal.

Strategy: A way to achieve objectives and ultimately goals. [Example: My 90-year-old mother did balance and leg-strengthening exercises (strategy), in order to be able to walk safely without her walker (objective), hoping that she could, at some point, go outside and take care of her plants (goal).]

Prioritization: Choosing strategies, objectives, or goals based upon their potential impact, achievability, importance, and/or perceived value.

Value: The major underlying reason for choosing and prioritizing particular goals, objectives, and strategies. An individual assessment of what is important or meaningful.

Preference: An individual's attitude towards various available options.

Risk Factor: An inherited or acquired attribute that increases the probability that a particular (usually undesirable) outcome will occur in the future.

Vulnerability: Susceptibility to a particular (usually undesirable) outcome as a result of one or more risk factors.

Resource: A personal attribute (e.g., intelligence, resilience), asset (e.g., knowledge, skill, money, insurance, time), or connection (e.g., family, friends) that can be used to achieve a desired outcome.

Investment: Personal stake in an (generally desired) outcome.

Obstacle: Something that gets in the way of the achievement of an objective or goal.

Challenge: Something that requires an investment of physical or mental effort, or a positive way to think of an obstacle.

Premature death: Death resulting from a preventable cause.

Premature disability: Disability resulting from a preventable cause.

Life expectancy: The average number of additional years a person or group of people is expected to live based upon their risk profile(s). Estimated life expectancy can be particularly helpful when prioritizing preventive strategies.

Health expectancy: The average number of additional years a person or group of people is expected to live free of significant disability based upon their risk profile(s).

Health-related quality of life: The degree and extent to which a person is able to comfortably participate in necessary, enjoyable, and meaningful life activities.

Meaningful life activity: An activity that gives life purpose or meaning.

Optimal growth and development: 1) Achievement of major developmental tasks; 2) development of resilience, adaptability, and the ability to handle challenges; 3) acquisition of the skills required to help others; and 4) progression through the levels of moral development.

A good death: A death that is 1) free from avoidable distress and suffering for the individual, their family, and caregivers; 2) in general accord with individual and family wishes; and 3) reasonably consistent with clinical, cultural, and ethical standards.

Interpersonal: Meaningful associations and interactions between people which impact the thoughts, feelings, and neurophysiology of those involved.

Same Words, Different Meanings

Some words are used in both problem-oriented and goal-oriented care, but the definitions are different as shown in the following table.

Table 13.1: Same words, different meanings

Word	Problem-Oriented Definition	Goal-Oriented Definition
Health	A state characterized by the absence of physical and psychological abnormalities; a point on a downward sloping curve.	The ability to fully experience and benefit from life's journey.
Health care	An applied scientific activity aimed at correcting or minimizing physical and psychological abnormalities in order to reduce their unwanted consequences.	A relationship-based support system intended to help patients clarify and achieve their personal goals using clinical methods.
Goal	Usually a measure related to an intermediate disease management outcome (e.g., a systolic BP < 140).	A desired outcome that can stand on its own merits. That is, it makes little sense to ask, "Why would you want that to happen?"
Risk factor	A characteristic, hazard, or behavior that increases the risk of an adverse health event.	A characteristic, hazard, or behavior that increases the risk of an adverse health event.
Death	The failure of medical care.	Life's final event.

Framing the Conversation

Mrs. Gooch, a 57-year-old African American mother of three and grandmother of six, had been a patient of mine for more than 10 years. Her medical diagnoses included diabetes, elevated blood pressure, and arthritis. During one of her office visits I said to her, "You seem to be enjoying life a lot," to which she replied that she was. I said, "I assume that one of the reasons you come in to see me is so I can help you stay alive as long as possible." Again, "Yes." Then I asked, "What would you still like to see and do before you die?"

She began to talk about her grandchildren, family gatherings, graduations, and marriages. I asked, "What do you think is the most important thing you could do, with my help, to increase the chance that you will live long enough to see those things happen?" She said, "I should probably stop smoking." When I strongly agreed, she said, "I'm going to do it," and she did.

Encouraging Mrs. Gooch to focus on her goals encouraged her to become invested in the strategies to achieve them. By "invested," I mean simply that Mrs. Gooch saw maximizing time with her family as important enough to make a significant investment of time and energy into smoking cessation. Within the problem-oriented framework, smoking would have been identified as one of Mrs. Gooch's problems, and she would have been advised to quit. For her, that had not been helpful.

The difference may seem subtle, but in my experience, it is huge. A goal-oriented approach ties the strategy — smoking cessation — to a meaningful personal goal – ability to participate in valued life activities. It frames the issue in positive (i.e., goal achievement) rather than negative (i.e., correcting an abnormality) terms. The positive approach is almost always more effective because it encourages patients to make a greater investment in their health. And greater investment nearly always leads to greater returns.

When I was first starting out in practice, I used to ask patients to tell me about themselves. While well intentioned, that question was much too broad and therefore of little value. Sometimes I would ask them how stressful their life was. I remember one particular young woman with terrible headaches who told me there was very little stress in her life. She said she had a good job, great marriage, nice house, and well-behaved kids. After several different headache medicines proved ineffective, I got a call from her husband. He began the conversation by admonishing me, "Do you have any idea how much stress my wife is under?" Then he proceeded to tell me.

After years of experience and a change in perspective, I found the quickest way to gain insight into a patient's life was to ask them to describe a typical day in their life. Some patients provided few details, while others gave a minute-by-minute account, but I was usually able to help them find the middle ground. "What time do you usually get up? Then what do you do? And after that?" Depending upon the challenges a patient was facing, it was usually helpful to further clarify some things. For example, "Why do you do it that way?" or "Do you have any trouble with that?" or "You didn't mention. . .(e.g., bathing, eating breakfast)."

After gaining some understanding of what a typical day is like, I learned to then ask, "What are the things that give you the most trouble?" and "What would you like to be able to do that you can't do now?" Notice I didn't ask, "What does your diabetes prevent you from doing?" or "What kinds of trouble does your arthritis cause you?" Those questions might be helpful for further clarification, but the main questions are about quality of life as a goal, unrelated to any specific health challenges. Once I established a longitudinal relationship with a patient, I would ask questions like, "For you, what activities and relationships make life worth living?" and "What conditions or circumstances would, for you, be worse than death?"

In my experience, those kinds of questions fit very comfortably into most clinical encounters and are well-received and even appreciated by patients. They certainly provide better information than the questions I tried years ago as a young, inexperienced physician, and they usually lead directly into discussions about goals, objectives, and strategies.

Discussing Options and Trade-Offs

After my prostatectomy for Stage B, localized prostate cancer, I had sensitive PSA tests every six months for two years to be sure all of the cancer had been removed. Since then, physicians have periodically asked me if I want to repeat that test to rule out metastatic disease. Because I have seen no evidence that treatment of metastatic prostate cancer is more effective if started prior to the onset of symptoms, I have always declined. If I were to develop symptoms suggestive of metastatic disease, I might agree to be tested, but I would have to be confident that treatment could increase my life expectancy significantly, and that the quality of life trade-offs would probably be worth it.

Most patients are hesitant to refuse tests and treatments recommended by their physicians. That is not surprising, since such decisions require knowledge of the pros and cons and probabilities associated with such decisions. Unfortunately, physicians too often lack this knowledge as well, and when they have it, they have difficulty providing it to patients. Recent efforts to create shared decision-making tools should be helpful.

What physicians and patients always underestimate are the adverse psychological effects and momentum for further testing and treatment created by a positive test result. Knowing that my PSA is elevated at this point would have a negative impact on my psyche with little or no increase in my life expectancy, but it would still be hard for me to refuse treatment. That is why the discussion of options and trade-offs needs to occur as early in the diagnostic or screening process as possible, ideally before the tests are ordered.

Traditional medical interventions like medications and procedures nearly always involve trade-offs, and those trade-offs should be discussed before a strategy is implemented. Depending on the patient's level of knowledge and interest, that conversation could be as simple as, "Is this something you are willing to do to live a little longer?" to "All medicines cause side effects. The side effects of this one are listed here. People who take this medicine once a day gain about one year of additional life on average, but some don't benefit at all and some gain more than that. Is this something you want to try?" Obviously, that requires physicians to have that kind of information available.

Trade-offs are particularly common near the end of life, when the gains in life expectancy often come at great cost in terms of quality of life. To make such decisions, patients need unbiased information and the recommendation of a respected and trusted professional. In my experience, it is almost always possible to present accurate information and a recommendation without unnecessarily eliminating hope, particularly if death is viewed as a natural part of life rather than an enemy to be defeated.

Chapter 14a

Helping Patients Build Physiologic Resilience

"That which does not kill us makes us stronger."
—Friedrich Nietzsche

RESILIENCE IS THE CAPACITY to successfully face challenges, overcome obstacles, and adapt to changing conditions. Physiological resilience depends upon optimally functioning biological processes and sufficient reserve capacity to allow us to survive periods of physiological stress and deprivation. And when physiological challenges are faced successfully, lasting improvements in function and greater resilience can result.

Resilience can be considered a goal - a version of becoming all you can be - or an objective along the path toward personal growth and development. When I was a teenager, I remember a debate I had with another boy my age during a Sunday School class over whether one should focus on helping others or on improving oneself. It took many years to me to figure out that the two are inextricably linked. Care for oneself is necessary if one is to help others, and helping others is a way to take care of oneself. Similarly, resilience is both a goal and an objective. In either case, it is unquestionably pertinent to health and therefore to health care.

By the way, it could also be argued that building resilience is really a strategy for achieving a longer, more enjoyable life and achieving a better death. That simply suggests that the four goals are not completely independent.

Use It or Lose It

To function properly, biological systems must be used. When I was a medical student long ago, we used three-hour glucose tolerance tests to diagnose diabetes mellitus. As a requirement for test accuracy, patients were required to consume sufficient carbohydrates for the three days prior to the test to make sure that their insulin response was fully activated. Scholastic Aptitude Test (SAT) scores tend to decline over time beyond high school graduation, not because of decreasing mental acuity, but because of lack of practice. Celibate nuns produce less vaginal mucous and are at greater risk of post-menopausal atrophic vaginal changes than sexually active women.

In a series of classic articles, Walter Bortz II, also mentioned in Chapter 1a, proposed that much of what we consider to be "normal aging" is actually *disuse*. He defined a *disuse syndrome* characterized by cardiovascular vulnerability, musculoskeletal fragility, metabolic instability, immunologic susceptibility, central nervous system compromise, and general frailty. By comparing oxygen delivery capacity (VO_2 max), in older athletes to those in sedentary people of the same age, he was able to show that fit 70-year-olds have the same capacity as sedentary 40-year-olds. That suggests that challenging physiological systems can make them stronger and potentially more resilient.

The following are some examples of how physicians can encourage people to become more resilient physiologically.

Immunity

We know a great deal about how the immune system develops and how it can be strengthened or weakened by the actions physicians and parents take. A critical factor during infancy involves the development of the intestinal microbiome. Bacteria begin to colonize the gut, skin, and oral and nasal cavities shortly after birth.

Gut-colonizing bacteria play a critical role in the development and modulation of both the humoral and cellular immune systems. Metabolites of micro-organisms signal cells of the innate immune system to respond to environmental threats, and disturbances of the intestinal biome can induce chronic inflammation and metabolic dysfunction. Normal exposure of infants to environmental bacteria seems to be helpful in this process and attempts to prevent such exposures through excessive cleanliness can be detrimental. Breastfeeding may also play a positive role, although the mechanisms are unclear. Once established, each person's microbiome is unique and relatively stable unless disturbed by disease, medications, toxins, or radical changes in diet.

Immunization is the most obvious example of a medical intervention that challenges a biological system, making it more resilient. During my time in West Africa, I had the opportunity to see far too many children die of measles pneumonia. There was an entire building devoted to the care and rehabilitation of polio victims. I was fortunate to only have to care for one patient with tetanus. My pre-travel typhoid and yellow fever immunizations no doubt protected me from those terrible diseases, which were all too common during my stay.

Throughout life, we are challenged by other pathogens for which immunizations are not available. In most cases, we respond by developing antibodies and cell-mediated immunity, making us less susceptible to future infections with those organisms. Early treatment with antibiotics can reduce or prevent this response and should therefore be avoided when possible. For example, delaying antibiotic treatment of bacterial middle ear infections for 5 days reduces the incidence of recurrent infections without increasing the risk of serious complications.

Muscle Strength

Resistance exercises increase the strength of muscles, and strong muscles can be protective during times of inactivity and injury. After a period of muscle inactivity (e.g. when immobilized in a cast), regaining lost strength takes four times as long as losing it. For reasons that are still unclear, it seems to take more and more exercise to maintain and build muscle strength as we age, especially beyond about age 75.

It is important to remember that exercises tend to be specific. Basketball does little to prepare one's musculoskeletal system for other sports like soccer. I prescribed leg lifts with weights to increase quadriceps strength in older people until it was discovered that back-against-the-wall squats are more helpful because they require synchronous use of all of the muscles required to rise from a chair. The same principle applies to other types of muscle strengthening exercises.

Strengthening muscles tends to require a minimum of two sets a day of at least ten repetitions against sufficient resistance that the last repetition of each set is somewhat difficult. Unfortunately, for reasons that are still unclear, it takes more exercise sets per day to maintain and build muscle strength as we age, especially beyond age 75.

Cardiopulmonary Resilience

Aerobic physical activity beyond the amount needed for survival builds cardiopulmonary resilience. Endurance training produces positive adaptive changes in heart size, heart rate, stroke volume, blood pressure, blood volume, and maximal oxygen uptake (VO2 max). That additional capacity can come in handy when facing a serious illness or injury.

Cognition

The onset of noticeable cognitive impairment in patients with dementia is delayed in individuals with higher educational attainment, and greater ongoing cognitive activity in work and leisure activities, suggesting that those modifiable factors contribute to cognitive resilience. Physical activity also increases levels of neural growth factor, which contributes to repair and regeneration of brain cells throughout life.

Balance

Balance is obviously critical to bipedal mobility. Falls and fear of falling are major causes of premature death and disability. It seems wise, therefore, to try to build resilience within the mechanisms involved in balance. Falling was a significant challenge for many of my geriatric patients. I often prescribed balance exercises beginning with tandem walking and balancing on each foot and progressing gradually to a balance board or referred them to physical therapy. Even patients with significant peripheral neuropathy were often able to increase their mobility and reduce their falls. We now know that one of the most effective ways to prevent falls is regular participation in Tai Chi. Yoga may also work. I prefer basketball and walking in the woods.

Physiologic Reserves

Each of our biological systems has a substantial amount of reserve capacity, which is rarely needed or used. That is why smokers often don't notice that they are losing pulmonary function until they are in pulmonary failure. Once those reserves are gone, the slope of the decline in function is steep. Part of my message to smokers who had signs of obstructive pulmonary disease but few symptoms was that they had probably used up all of their extra lung capacity and were living at the edge of a cliff — which I drew for them. I pointed out that loss of any more lung tissue could result in the need for continuous home oxygen therapy.

Reserve capacity becomes extremely important during times of physiological stress. Reserve capacity also tends to diminish with increasing age. It makes sense for us to encourage patients to build and protect functional reserve capacities, but, for most of our body systems, we don't know much about how to do that.

An exception is bone mineral density. Peak bone strength appears to be dependent upon both physical activity and calcium intake during childhood, and especially during adolescence when most bone mineral deposition occurs. Weight-bearing activities throughout life build additional bone strength, which comes in handy when bone loss begins to happen after menopause and with aging.

Many vitamins and minerals are stored in our bodies for later use. Protein is stored in muscle. Energy is stored primarily as fat. When we are sick, we need more nutrients, but we often don't feel like eating. Nutritional reserves then become essential. When we recover, we overeat for a while to restock.

Diet diary studies have found that the diets of most people over the age of 75 include inadequate amounts of a number of micronutrients. Those dietary inadequacies rarely cause clinical signs or symptoms in the absence of physiological stress. Older people have a harder time both building reserves and restocking after illnesses. In one classic nursing home study, malnutrition was more strongly associated with number of hospitalizations than with current nutritional intake.

In addition to encouraging all people to eat a well-balanced diet, we should encourage those at risk for nutritional deficiencies to build up their reserves of both macro- and micro-nutrients. That will often require vitamin/mineral and/or protein/calorie supplements. Older patients in particular should also be advised to take protein/calorie/vitamin/mineral nutritional supplements (e.g., Ensure, Boost) for several weeks following episodes of illness.

Vital Organs

I feel obliged to say a few words about several under-appreciated organs. Laurence J. Peter is credited with having said, "A doctor is a person who still has his adenoids, tonsils, and appendix."

The *tonsils and adenoids* are the first line of defense against respiratory pathogens in childhood with some role in shaping the adaptive immune system. Early tonsillectomy/adenoidectomy is associated with an *increased* incidence of otitis and sinusitis and with subsequent development of asthma and other allergic conditions.

The *gall bladder* releases bile into the small intestine at just the right times to maximize digestion of fats. Cholecystectomy alters the intestinal microbiome and is associated with an increased incidence of colorectal cancer.

The *appendix* is an immunologically active organ and a reservoir for helpful intestinal microbes. Removal is associated with higher rates of recurrence of C. difficile gastroenteritis and possibly with Parkinson's Disease.

The *uterus and ovaries* continue to be active components of the endocrine system even after menopause. Hysterectomy without ovariectomy is associated with increases in weight, blood pressure, and lipids, and increased rates of coronary artery disease and heart failure. Ovariectomy is epidemiologically associated with an increased long-term risk of Parkinsonism, cognitive impairment, anxiety, depression, and premature mortality.

Chapter 14b

Helping Patients Build Psychological Resilience

"Life course planning in America is common in the financial planning arena, but has not been applied in the same way to lifelong improvement of self-care competency, and planning for learning the skills of relationships, care receiving, and caregiving. Thus, many older people are not prepared for the natural occurrences of physical decline, loss, and grief."

—Jill A. Bennett, PhD, RN and

Marna K. Flaherty Robb, RN, MSN

"What happens to us becomes part of us. Resilient people do not bounce back from hard experiences; they find healthy ways to integrate them into their lives. In time, people find that great calamity met with great spirit can create great strength."

—Eric Greitens

PSYCHOLOGICAL RESILIENCE HAS BEEN DEFINED by the American Psychological Association (APA) as "the process of adapting well in the face of adversity, trauma, tragedy, threats, or significant sources of stress—such as family and relationship problems, serious health problems, or workplace and financial stressors." The APA goes on to state that psychological resilience is not a trait that people have or don't have, but a set of behaviors, thoughts, and actions that can be learned and developed by anyone. Physicians are in a position to help patients develop psychological resilience through education, support, empathy, encouragement, counseling, reframing, personal example, and referral.

Most of the evidence-based strategies for building psychological resilience are related to the three essential psychological requirements identified by Edward Deci and Richard Ryan: relatedness, autonomy, and competence as shown in the following table.

Table 14b.1 Strategies for Building Psychological Resilience

Essential Psychological Needs	Strategies for Building Resilience
Relatedness / Connection	1. Develop good relationships with key family members, friends, and others. 2. Accept help and support from those who care about you. 3. Be active in civic, religious, or other social groups. 4. Cultivate feelings of universal connectedness through faith, meditation, exposure to nature, etc.
Autonomy	1. Take decisive actions on adverse situations rather than avoiding or detaching from them. 2. Develop realistic goals and do something regularly to move toward those goals. 3. Avoid seeing crises as insurmountable problems. Reframe them as challenges.
Competence	1. Look for opportunities for self-discovery, particularly in the face of losses, tragedies, and other hardships. 2. Nurture a positive view of your ability to solve problems and trust your instincts. 3. Focus on sources of personal strength and successful strategies used in the past.

Building Psychological Resilience in Childhood

A goal of all parents should be to raise resilient children who will be able to successfully face the challenges they are likely to face throughout life.

Attachment and Trust

Development of trust is the first and most important developmental task. It requires the presence of a dependable, responsive person with whom the infant can develop a secure attachment. When such a person is unreliable, unresponsive, or absent, the child is likely to have trouble forming healthy relationships and dealing with losses throughout life. The impact of a dependable attachment figure during early childhood on psychological resilience can be profound, and there are no consistently effective remedies for its absence. Physicians and society as a whole should do everything possible to encourage the development of caring relationships between infants and one or more adults during the first three years of life.

Positive Parenting

In *Outliers*, Malcolm Gladwell summarizes research done in California in which a large cohort of children with very high IQs were followed for several decades. According to Gladwell, the researchers found that success in life was more likely when a person's IQ was at least 130, but, above that, IQ was unrelated to future success. In children with IQs greater than 130, the difference between success and failure was determined by parenting. Children who had been taught by their parents to view obstacles as surmountable challenges were more likely to succeed than those whose parents failed to instill that attitude.

Self-made billionaire inventor of Spanx, Sara Blakely, when asked about the most important advice she ever received, told how, as a child, her father taught her to celebrate her failures. Each week he would ask her, "What did you fail at this week?" When she told him, he would give her a high-five. Teaching children to view negative experiences as opportunities to learn and grow is one of the greatest gifts a parent, teacher, or physician can give.

Based upon an analysis of data from the 2016 and 2017 National Survey of Children's Health, greater family resilience and connection was associated with children's interest and curiosity in learning new things, persistence in completing tasks, and capacity to regulate emotions. Indeed, family resilience mitigated some of the adverse consequences of adverse childhood events, inadequate household income, and health challenges. In another study, greater resilience in adolescents with chronic musculoskeletal pain was associated with less pain and disability and with greater energy and better health-related quality of life.

Resiliency Training Exercises

As our understanding of the importance of psychological resilience has grown, a variety of resiliency training programs have been developed for children, adolescents, and adults. Most are based upon the following individual attributes and skills that have been found by researchers to be associated with resilience:

- Social competence,
- Problem-solving skills,
- Sense of autonomy, self-efficacy, and goal-setting,
- Sense of purpose, hope, or meaning,
- Stress management, and
- Cognitive reframing.

Most of these programs use strength-based as opposed to deficit-reduction approaches. In educational settings these programs are sometimes called "social and emotional learning (SEL) curricula." A well-known set of resiliency training exercises is the *Teen Resiliency-Building Workbook* developed by Ed Liptak and Ester Leutenberg, which is available to parents.

In a randomized controlled trial, the Promoting Resilience in Stress

Management intervention (PRISM-P), when delivered to the parents of children with cancer, improved the parents' self-reported resilience and benefit-finding skills.

Building Psychological Resilience in Adults

The Chronic Disease Self-Management Program developed by Kate Lorig and her research team at Stanford, now available to patients throughout the country through state departments of health, involves patients with chronic health challenges in six weekly 90-minute interactive workshops designed to build self-confidence, improve decision-making, and facilitate realistic goal-setting. The groups typically meet in various community settings, such as senior centers, churches, and hospitals. Each group is facilitated by two trained leaders from organizations licensed to provide the program. Documented short-term benefits include increased energy, reduced pain, increased physical activity, improved mood, and better communication with physicians.

Coleman and colleagues at the University of Colorado developed an effective multifaceted intervention to reduce hospital readmission rates, which they have called The Care Transitions Intervention (CTI). Central to their approach are trained and certified health coaches whose task is to help patients improve their ability to advocate for themselves and become more confident in their problem-solving skills. A post-discharge home visit is used to encourage patients to acquire the skills required for them to participate in their care more effectively.

Another version of health coaching, called "capacity coaching," has been adapted for use with complex patients. It is based upon the premise that there are five major factors that determine patients' capacity to cope with multiple health challenges: Biography, Resources, Environment, accomplishing Work, and Social (BREWS). Coaching strategies are designed to address each of those factors.

Buddhism and Resilience

Buddhism provides guidance about how to deal with the realities of life through psychological resilience. It is based upon the following observations or "truths" about life: that suffering is inevitable; it often results from our attachment to particular outcomes; and there are ways to reduce its psychological impact, in part by recognizing that everything changes over time. Those observations suggest a variety of actions that people can take to achieve resilience.

- Avoid becoming too attached to a particular outcome. It is okay to prefer that things work out in a certain way, but it can be hazardous to become addicted to it.
- View losses as things you had for a time, rather than things you have lost.
- Find a meaningful purpose in life that can help you view both positive and negative events as opportunities for growth (e.g., to make the world a better place or to become a better person).
- Avoid blame and negative judgments. Assume that everyone is doing the best they can, given their background and circumstances. Practice forgiveness of self and others.
- Try to find joy and humor in all things. Practice smiling.
- Find colleagues and mentors who provide psychological support by helping you self-reflect, debrief, and validate.
- Incorporate reflection and reappraisal in everyday life. Avoid catastrophizing. Learn to ask, "Is it really so?"
- View the inevitability of change as a gift. Each new day brings with it an opportunity to change our view and our responses to suffering.
- Learn to accept support from others so that they have the opportunity to benefit from the joy of giving.
- Cultivate joy by wishing others well.
- Practice meditation, which strengthens the inner resources that

give us confidence to deal with the ups and downs of life.

- Practice mindfulness — conscious awareness of the present moment. Mindfulness Based Stress Reduction (MBSR) training is available in many locations.

What Physicians Can Do

Opportunities to help patients become more resilient often occur while discussing other goals, obstacles, and challenges. I recall, for example, a patient who had been admitted to my inpatient rehabilitation service following a left hemispheric stroke. Over the course of his rehabilitation program, I helped him reconceptualize the event as "the biggest challenge you have ever faced," and we were able to generate optimism by reviewing how well he had managed to face prior challenges in his life. The rehabilitation setting naturally supported his needs for relationship, autonomy, and competence. The staff psychologist also taught him relaxation and mindfulness techniques. His mood quickly improved, and he did well.

Physicians can pass along the suggestions from this chapter at opportune moments during visits, post them on the practice web page, print them on appointment reminder cards, or frame them to hang in the waiting room and exam rooms. They can be used to help patients view their situations differently. Parents and adult patients can be referred to the resources and training opportunities mentioned.

Chapter 15

Physician Responsibilities

"Clinicians, anyone honored by the possibility to care, must notice and act toward each person in need of their care. They must appreciate each person's circumstance, concerns, contexts, biology, and biography. To appreciate each patient, the clinician must throw moorings that, for the moment, partner the boats."

—Victor Montori, MD

"A physician who merely spreads an array of vendibles in front of the patient, and then says, 'Go ahead and choose. It's your life,' is guilty of shirking his duty, if not of malpractice. The physician, to be sure, should list the alternatives and describe their pros and cons, but then, instead of asking the patient to make the choice, the physician should recommend a course of action."

—Franz J. Ingelfinger, M.D.

UPON READING DRAFTS OF THE CHAPTERS in this book, my wife expressed concern that I am expecting too much of physicians. While I agree that I am challenging physicians to think harder and invest more in the outcomes of their patients, I don't think that is too much to ask, given the intellectual, emotional, and financial rewards. In fact, I think physicians, particularly primary care physicians, who practice goal-oriented care are generally more satisfied and less likely to burn out than those who practice problem-oriented care. The following are some of the responsibilities of physicians practicing goal-oriented care.

Know Clinical Medicine

To an even greater extent than problem-oriented physicians, goal-oriented physicians need to know how the human body works, what can go wrong with it, and what can be done when that happens. When the focus is on patient-relevant outcomes, it is not sufficient to be able to make a correct diagnosis and look up its treatment. It is important to understand the underlying risk factors, natural history, pathophysiological changes, and potential consequences of treatment.

A legitimate concern of physicians who implement goal-oriented care is that while focusing on patient goals, potentially life-limiting conditions might be missed. That shouldn't happen if there is a method for systematically looking for such conditions, for example by conducting annual comprehensive histories and physical examinations. The difference between goal-oriented and problem-oriented care is that in goal-oriented care the search for abnormalities is viewed as a preventive strategy. Identified conditions are considered risk factors, part of the overall risk profile for each patient.

Mrs. Kinasewitz was a 67-year-old widow who, while on vacation, developed a cardiac arrhythmia requiring an overnight hospitalization. At discharge, she was told to see a physician as soon as possible after arriving home. Her daughter, who was an outreach coordinator at our medical center, brought her to see me as a new patient. Her complete medical, family, and social history were unremarkable aside from some mild intermittent asthma and a history of a hysterectomy for fibroids a decade earlier. On physical examination, I noticed a small scar above her right clavicle. When I asked her about it, she recalled having had an abnormal chest X-ray prior to her hysterectomy, which led to a biopsy of some lymph nodes in her chest. She was told that she had evidence of sarcoidosis, but that it didn't appear to be active and would probably never cause her any problems.

Having just read a review article in *The New England Journal of Medicine*, I knew that cardiac sarcoidosis could cause fatal arrhythmias and was usually discovered post-mortem. A thallium scan, serum ACE level and sedimentation rate confirmed the diagnosis of cardiac sarcoidosis, and, after consultation with both a cardiologist and a pulmonologist, in the absence of evidence-based guidelines, Mrs. K, her daughter, and I decided on treatment with high-dose corticosteroids. The treatment worked. Her sarcoidosis, which was also present in her lungs and may have contributed to her wheezing, regressed. We were able to eventually taper the corticosteroid dosage, and she did well for a number of years thereafter, with no further arrhythmias.

Learn How to Apply Clinical Evidence to Individual Patients

In part to make results look more impressive, researchers usually report the effect of interventions as relative risk reductions (RRR) and relative reductions in mortality rates. For example, statins can reduce the risk of adverse cardiovascular events by 20 - 25% per 40mg/dl reduction in LDL cholesterol in at-risk patients with no history of atherosclerotic cardiovascular disease. All-cause mortality rate is reduced by as much as 10%. To translate those estimates into numbers meaningful to individual patients, it is necessary to calculate absolute risk reductions (ARR; ARR = Baseline Risk X RRR X 100%). That often requires going back to the published articles to find pretreatment risk or risk in the comparison group.

For example, if a cholesterol-lowering medication can reduce the risk of an MI by 25% and the MI rate in the comparison group was 20%, then the drug lowered the risk of MI for the average patient by 5% (0.25 X 0.20 X 100%). It may also be necessary to further adjust the ARR estimate to make it consistent with the goal (e.g., prevention of premature death or disability). Depending upon how MIs were detected in the study, the percentage of MIs that resulted in death or disability was probably lower than 100%, so the ARR for death or disability was less than 5%. Because goal-oriented preventive care involves prioritization, these probability estimates can be important.

When I was first advised by my primary care physician to take a statin, I had reservations. So I asked him to help me calculate the predicted benefit. Based upon the calculator available at that time, my 10-year risk of an MI was 12%. Assuming an RRR of 25%, taking a statin could be expected to lower my 10-year MI risk to 9%, (12% - [0.25 X 0.12 X 100%]), a reduction in risk of 3%. Assuming that two-thirds of MIs cause death or long-term disability, the probability of actual benefit was 2%. I decided instead to increase my level of physical activity and improve my diet.

Notice that no information was available regarding how many weeks, months, or years of life I could expect to gain or how many fewer weeks, months, or years of disability I could avoid by taking a statin. Those patient-relevant estimates are rarely calculable from published studies.

Build Strong Clinical Relationships

Therapeutic physician-patient relationships are based upon mutual respect and trust. One of the most important responsibilities of physicians is to have and demonstrate unconditional positive regard for every patient. My mother taught me to assume that all human beings are doing their best, given their circumstances. Experience has taught me that, true or not, that perspective is extremely helpful. Patients' respect for and trust in a physician is built over time upon the physician's competence, reliability, and sincerity.

Nearly as important for goal-oriented care are the relationships among team members within the practice. Teamwork requires dedicated time for training, practice, and reflection, which can occur during daily huddles, weekly staff meetings, and annual practice retreats. The best way to ensure that these strategies are effective is to focus them on the goals of each individual patient. Research has shown goal concordance to be the key to effective teamwork within health care organizations. A goal-oriented approach is easier to implement in settings in which mental health care and rehabilitative services, particularly occupational and physical therapists, are members of the primary care team.

Relationships with individual patients are enhanced by relationships with family members and other caregivers. The relationship a practice has with its patients can also be enhanced by encouraging patients to be involved in practice quality improvement efforts. That can be accomplished in a number of ways, but the trend is for practices to create patient advisory councils.

Also important are relationships with outside medical consultants. Now that most primary care physicians spend less time in hospitals, continuing education conferences and social gatherings have become more important for this purpose. It is also critical to choose consultants who will provide telephonic or secure e-mail consultations.

Establish a Collaborative Process

Carl Rogers, father of client-centered therapy, after carefully studying the therapeutic features of psychological counseling, concluded that the three clinician skills primarily responsible for positive changes were congruence (genuineness, openness, authenticity), unconditional positive regard, and accurate empathic responses. There is little doubt that these skills apply equally well to medical encounters.

In her book *Patient-Centered Medicine: Transforming the Clinical Method*, Dr. Moira Stewart and her co-authors describe an approach to clinical encounters that encourages patients to express their concerns and objectives. The acronym she uses is BATHE: background, affect, trouble, handling, and empathy. For example, a physician might ask her patient to explain the reason for the visit, whether and how it has affected the patient emotionally, what trouble it has caused in their life, and how well they are handling the situation. The physician could then respond to that information empathically (e.g., "That must be frustrating." Or "You feel angry because...")

As described earlier in this book, my approach was to discuss current health concerns within the context of a typical day and as events within the patient's life story. When possible, I also found it helpful to establish a relationship with each patient's family health expert, the relative everyone in the family goes to for health advice. When that wasn't possible, I asked patients to tell me how that person felt about the decisions we were making.

Support Patients' Psychological Needs

People do better when their basic psychological needs are met. If you use goal-oriented care principles and techniques, that should be virtually automatic. However, as with all skills, there are nuances. The physician-patient relationship is key to therapeutic effectiveness. While it requires an intellectual and emotional investment from both parties, it is a professional relationship limited in breadth to health-related matters. From the primary care physician, in addition to professional competence, it requires accessibility, a longitudinal commitment, diligence, honesty, and the willingness to be an advocate for the patient within the health care system.

Physicians can support patients' autonomy need by genuinely valuing their information and input and by respecting their decisions. It is helpful to remember that physicians are consultants. It is up to our patients to make nearly all health care decisions in consultation with us and whoever else they trust to guide them. As autonomy is threatened by old age and infirmity, it is especially important that physicians advocate for their patients' right to make autonomous choices until they are no longer capable of doing so.

In my geriatric practice, patients often insisted on remaining in their homes beyond the point of safety, requiring family members to come to assist and sometimes rescue them. It was my practice to tell my patients that I was their advocate and would support them in whatever decision they made as long as they had weighed the impact of that decision on family and friends.

As patients successfully face challenges, overcome obstacles, and make progress toward their goals, it is the responsibility of their physicians to congratulate them, reinforcing their feelings of competence. When new challenges arise, it is often helpful to remind patients of the challenges they have successfully faced in the past.

Help Patients Tell Their Stories

Human beings organize thoughts and memories within stories. Helping patients tell their stories is therefore extremely important. When a physician or team member helps a patient organize the events of their life chronologically, they can more clearly see trajectory they are on and make better decisions about whether and how to make adjustments if necessary They can also be encouraged to question assumptions and to look at challenges in different ways. This approach need not consume additional time for at least two reasons. It would be done instead of rather than in addition to problem-oriented history-taking, and it can be accomplished over time.

To hear and understand a patient's story, one must be fully present. Aside from brief note-taking if necessary, it is not a time for clicking through an electronic record or attempting to fully document the encounter. I recognize that such documentation is necessary, and that it takes time. The best solution I have seen to date is the use of scribes. The cost of a scribe is roughly equivalent to the revenue generated from seeing one more patient each half day. That seems to me to be a price worth paying.

Understanding a patient's story requires understanding the major characters, including of course the patient (personality style, views on health and health care, decision-making process, and values), and members of the patient's family and social network. Particularly important are those people who help the patient face major challenges.

It is also important to understand the feelings expressed in each patient's story and to state or otherwise acknowledge them. Empathic statements can take the following form: "You are/were feeling <...> because <...>." Adding a goal-relevant statement to the end of such a sentence can also be helpful, such as, "and you would like to <...>".

Because physicians are often involved in the major life events that can alter the course of patients' lives, and because of the experience gained from watching others go through similar challenges, we can play a critical role in helping patients make wise choices at those times. In fact, this is one of our most important responsibilities: to encourage patients not to withdraw from life, alienate key family members, become addicted to drugs, unhealthy behaviors, or unrealistic expectations, or adopt a sick role.

The tools of narrative medicine fit nicely within the framework of goal-oriented care. Narrative medicine, as described in Rita Charon's pioneering book, *The Principles and Practice of Narrative Medicine*, is "medicine practiced with the competence to recognize, absorb, interpret, and be moved by the stories of illness." Using literary skills, doctors can learn to analyze patients' stories, providing insights into who they are and how they arrived at that point in their lives, and also educate, and help them face health challenges of life, illness, and death.

Help Patients Develop Resources

We all have risk factors and vulnerabilities, but equally important are the resources patients have to face challenges, overcome obstacles, and reduce risks. Key among these are health literacy, fund of medical knowledge, family and social support, and physical and psychological resilience. Assessment of resources can be accomplished during wellness visits and, over time, during routine encounters.

Every visit is educational. It is the physician's responsibility to make sure that what is taught and learned is helpful. When health challenges are chronic, patients should be encouraged to become experts on their conditions. When health challenges are recurrent, patients need to be better prepared to handle subsequent episodes. The educational assistance provided should be tied to each patient's goals whenever possible.

Humans learn as much from what is done as from what is said. For example, research has shown that when patients are given prescriptions for antibiotics for self-limited infections, the lesson they may learn is that they should have come in earlier.

Make Professional Recommendations

Presenting patients with options and letting them choose is insufficient. Patients expect and deserve a professional opinion. That opinion should be based not on what the physician would do but on what the physician believes would be in the best interest of the patient, given their values, goals, preferences, resources, and limitations. This is particularly important when the patient can no longer participate in decision-making and family members must become involved, for example when the patient is seriously ill. The following is the approach I used in such situations.

I invited all those with information bearing on pending decisions to meet. I explained that the purpose of the meeting was to share information about the patient's medical situation and previously stated values and preferences so that we could make the best possible decisions on their behalf. At the beginning of the meeting I emphasized that I wanted to be sure the pending medical decisions were consistent with the patient's prior expressed values and preferences. After explaining the patient's medical situation and the decisions that needed to be made, I asked those in attendance what, if anything, they knew about the patient's values and preferences as they might pertain to the current situation. Sometimes I would ask more specifically about meaningful life activities and conditions worse than death. Once all of the information was "on the table," I summarized it and made a recommendation, explaining my reasons. I then asked the family to react to my recommendations. In most cases, families agreed with my recommendations.

Of course, patients and family members don't always agree with professional recommendations. In such situations, it is important to identify the person with the legal authority to make the decision.

Employ Effective Therapeutic Strategies

While we have a responsibility to provide advice, advice-giving turns out to be less effective than other therapeutic strategies listed below.

- Acceptance and validation
- Empathic responses
- Positive expectations
- Encouragement
- Praise
- Supportive listening and strategic questioning
- Reassurance
- Education
- Advocacy
- Reframing
- Assisted reminiscence
- Normalization
- Role modeling

Collect and Manage Information

It is the responsibility of physicians to record the information and thought processes used in health care decision-making. To my knowledge, no physician has ever been successfully sued after having documented a reasonable decision-making process that involved collecting relevant facts, engaging in a collaborative discussion with the patient, and making reasonable strategic decisions. Documentation is particularly important in goal-oriented care when physicians and patients may be more likely to choose to deviate from population-based guidelines.

Current electronic record systems make it difficult to record the information important for goal-oriented care. I suggest finding somewhere in the record to create a Patient Profile that includes information about quality of life priorities. Ideally this profile should appear whenever the record is opened or at least when a new note is started. There also needs to be a place to document conditions viewed as worse than death, preferences regarding end-of-life care, and contact information for surrogate decision-makers.

At this point it probably makes sense to include as many risk factors as possible in the Problem List. That would need to include social, environmental, and behavioral risk factors as well as conditions traditionally thought of as diseases. If it is possible, I suggest putting the most important risk factors for future death and disability at the top of the list. The only places I can think of to put information about resilience are in the Patient Profile and Past History sections. I suggest noting who the "family health expert" is in the Family History section.

As discussed earlier, goal-oriented care requires that referral and consultation letters be more precise, including both what is requested and how that relates to the patient's goals.

Provide Wisdom and Perspective

Since people are inclined to focus on current quality of life concerns, an important responsibility of physicians is to make sure they also think about prevention and end-of-life planning. This can be as simple as making sure all patients schedule regular wellness visits that include end-of-life discussions. It is also important to help patients view their health challenges within the broader context of their life stories, creating a logical transition to discussions of prevention and end-of-life values and preferences.

Chapter 16

Making the Transition:
A 12-Step Program

"Physicians think they do a lot for a patient when they give his disease a name."

—Immanuel Kant

"We shall have to learn to refrain from doing things just because we know how to do them."

—Theodore Fox

BECAUSE OF THE ENVIRONMENTS in which we were trained and practice, it is hard to make the shift from problem-oriented to goal-oriented thinking. I suggest you proceed in steps, from easiest to most difficult. Take enough time to master each step before moving to the next one.

Step 1: Establish Simple Processes and Habits

- Establish annual wellness visits focused on life extension and advanced care planning with homework assigned prior to the visit that includes:
  * Identification of risk factors, risk mitigation efforts, vulnerabilities, and resources (Appendix A); and
  * Clarification of end-of-life care values and preferences, and completion of advance directive documents (Appendix B).
- Use the above information to shape discussions with patients to de-

velop rational, acceptable, prioritized prevention plans, considering most likely causes of death and future disability.

- Routinely incorporate the following questions into non-wellness encounters:
  * What is a typical day like for you? Walk me through your day.
  * Which daily activities give you the most trouble?
  * What else would you like to be able to do that you can't do now?
- View every encounter as an educational opportunity. Most health challenges are chronic or recurrent. Teach patients what they need to know to prevent and mitigate future occurrences.

Step 2: Cultivate Key Professional Relationships

- Identify local well-trained physical and occupational therapists, learn more about what they can offer your patients, and cultivate professional relationships with them.
- Identify a local podiatrist who is skilled in both therapeutic and preventive strategies.
- Identify accessible mental health professionals whose skills include motivational interviewing, cognitive behavioral therapy, and behavior modification, and cultivate strong professional relationships with them.
- Identify attorneys who specialize in end-of-life planning and establish professional relationships with them.

Step 3: Develop Staff Training, Patient Education, and Clinical Support Tools

- Develop a goal-oriented care training program for staff.
- Develop goal-oriented patient education materials focused on prevention and/or mitigation of recurrent health challenges (e.g., URIs, low back pain, migraines, etc.). (Appendix C)
- Develop and use clinical decision support tools relevant to preven-

tion (e.g., life expectancy tables, impact of various preventive measures on life expectancy, times required to benefit from various screening tests). (Appendix D)

- Develop and implement processes for routinely assessing the effects of quality of life strategies (e.g., symptom diaries, periodic drug holidays, N-of-1 protocols).

Step 4: Learn to Use the Threshold Principle and Law of Diminishing Returns

- Remember that multiple factors contribute to nearly every health challenge. Practice helping patients make lists of the factors that could be contributing to their most difficult challenges. Then teach them how addressing as many of those factors as possible might get them below the threshold for symptoms even if the main cause can't be eliminated. Begin with the most obvious one.

Headaches

Nearly everyone is susceptible to migraine headaches. Those who have frequent migraines are simply closer to the migraine threshold. While a genetic predisposition cannot currently be altered, many other contributing factors can be. Some of the many factors that can contribute to migraines are listed in Table 17.1. Even if eliminating one of them is ineffective, eliminating several of them simultaneously can be. A migraine diary can be very helpful. It is important to remember, however, that the effects of triggers are not always immediate. Headaches can occur days after exposure.

- Try not to ask patients to do too many things at once. Help them prioritize. Suggest they try to implement one or a few doable strategies at a time before adding additional ones. Help them pick strategies likely to have the greatest impact on goal achievement.

Table 16.1. Factors Known to Contribute to Migraines

Contributing Factors	Examples
Emotional/Behavioral	Fatigue; Lack of sleep or altered sleep pattern; Emotional stress; Hunger; Overexertion
Environmental	Loud noises; Bright lights; Excessive motion; Strong smells; Painful stimuli (e.g., neck injury, temporomandibular joint problems, sinus inflammation); Changes in weather (e.g., barometric pressure, humidity, temperature)
Dietary	Fermented foods (e.g., red wine, aged cheeses, yeast in fresh bread and yogurt); Foods containing caffeine, MSG, or nitrates (e.g., coffee, chocolate, Chinese food, processed meats); Prepackaged/prepared foods (e.g., TV dinners, frozen meals, pizza, macaroni and cheese); Foods containing hydrolyzed protein products (e.g., canned soups); Pickled, preserved, or marinated foods (e.g., olives, pickles, sauerkraut); Peanuts; Aspartame; Beans, peas, and lentils; Onions; Certain fruits (e.g., bananas, citrus, raisins, red plums, papayas, passion fruit)
Hormonal	Reduced estrogen levels (e.g., premenstrual, post-menopausal)
Medications	Proton pump inhibitors Overuse of pain medications and triptans

Step 5: Develop and Implement Clinical Pathways

- Establish clinical pathways to help patients make critical behavior changes. Begin with the most common and challenging preventive strategies encountered in your practice (Appendix E). Note: Addiction-related pathways will probably require developing professional relationships with Quit Lines, addiction counselors, and Alcoholics Anonymous and Narcotics Anonymous members willing to take phone calls from patients during primary care clinical encounters.

Step 6: Learn How to Support Personal Growth and Development

- Spend some time reviewing developmental stages across the lifespan and the challenges associated with their achievement. *(https://en.wikibooks.org/wiki/ Human_Physiology/ Development:_birth_through_death).(https:// www.goodtherapy.org/ blog/psychpedia/erikson-eight-stages-development).*
- Review the principles and clinical applications of Self Determination Theory.
- Investigate locally available resiliency training programs as well as opportunities for learning mindfulness, yoga, Tai Chi, and meditation.

Step 7: Reduce your Use of Diagnostic Labels

- Learn to use diagnostic labels only when their use is likely to help patients achieve their goals, recognizing the potential for adverse effects. Focus first on health challenges that have been arbitrarily dichotomized.

Attention Deficit Hyperactivity Disorder (ADHD)

Most vulnerabilities and risk factors have greater relevance in some settings than in others. ADHD is a good example. Nearly all children, especially boys, have some trouble paying attention and sometimes act impulsively. Such behaviors are relevant only when they interfere with quality of life or success in school since education reduces premature death and disability. The diagnosis of ADHD is often based upon subjective test scores above a certain arbitrary cut-point.

Giving a child or adult the label, ADHD, may be helpful when services (e.g., additional teaching assistance) or other benefits (e.g., medications) depend upon doing so. However, labeling alters the child's self-perception and the perceptions of family members, teachers, and others toward that child in ways that can be either positive or negative. Labeling results in a tendency to pigeonhole the child, blaming all behaviors and challenges on ADHD. The ADHD label can also be self-fulfilling, leading teachers to look for aberrant behavior and children to then over-exhibit it. Determining when to use the ADHD label requires clinical judgment and an understanding of the child, family, and situation.

Blood Pressure

It is worth remembering that blood pressure is a continuous measure, which has been dichotomized for purposes of distinguishing "normal" from "abnormal." The adverse effects of diagnostic labeling have been particularly well-documented for hypertension. Clearly some patients feel less healthy after they are told they have a named disorder like hypertension. The alternative to the standard approach is to simply refer to it as "your blood pressure," and to discuss lowering it as one way to increase life expectancy and reduce future disability.

As a risk factor, blood pressure is composed of at least four different interrelated values: systolic pressure, diastolic pressure, mean arterial pressure (MAP), and pulse pressure (PP). One or more of those parameters are associated with at least four common adverse events: stroke (CVA), heart attack (MI), heart failure (CHF), and chronic kidney disease (CKD). As with some other cardiovascular risk reduction strategies, BP reduction probably has at least two separate beneficial effects. It reduces ongoing stress and damage to the heart and arterial system, and it reduces the risk of acute plaque rupture and embolization from atherosclerotic arteries. Until all of this complexity can be further unraveled, it is probably best to focus on systolic BP as the best single predictor of adverse events, recognizing that it may actually represent both a risk factor, particularly in younger people, and a consequence, particularly in older people, of progressive atherosclerosis.

Lowering BP population-wide would save tens of thousands of lives and prevent countless disabling strokes and heart attacks each year. However, the benefits for individuals are much less impressive, they take years to achieve, and some people derive great benefits while others derive practically none. It is important to recommend BP reduction to those most likely to benefit. That requires more knowledge and thought than simply treating everyone to the same target.

The decision regarding whether to suggest BP reduction hinges on the patient's current systolic BP, their short- and long-term risk of a cardiovascular event, other cardiovascular risk reduction options available to them, and their ability and willingness to do what it would take to lower their BP for long periods of time. For some outcomes like CHF and possibly CVA, the impact of BP reduction will likely be greater per mmHg at higher initial BPs. That is, lowering systolic BP from 200 to 180 may have a greater impact on risk than lowering it from 160 to 140. For others, like MI, the impact curve is probably lower and flatter. However, the data needed to prove this are only available from risk prediction tools like David Eddy's Archimedes prediction model.

Average risk reduction estimates from clinical trials are shown below. In those trials, the average systolic BP difference between intervention and control groups was 10 to 15 mmHg.

Table 16.2. Average Five-Year Risk Reduction
Estimates from Clinical Trials of BP

Risk Parameter	CVA	MI	CHF	All-Cause Mortality
RRR/5yrs.	35%	25%	50%	13%
ARR/5yr. if risk is 2%/yr.	3.5% (10% to 6.5%)	2.5% (10% to 7.5%)	5% (10% to 5%)	1.8% (10% to 8.2%)

RRR = relative risk reduction
ARR = absolute risk reduction

Lowering systolic blood pressure below 140 in patients at risk for adverse cardiovascular events has been shown to reduce the occurrence of cardiovascular events from 2.19% to 1.65% (ARR = 0.54%/year), but it also increased the risk of serious adverse events like syncope, electrolyte abnormalities, and acute renal injury.

The most accurate methods for measuring BP are multiple automated BP readings in the office and 24-hour BP monitoring at home. The accuracy of non-automated BP measurements by a nurse, MA, or clinician can be improved by proper patient positioning (sitting with feet on the floor, arm supported at heart level, first measurement discarded). The same applies to non-automated home BP measurements.

As stated earlier, most people could derive some benefit from lowering their BP to just above syncopal levels. Their hearts and arteries would last longer. However, reducing BP over long periods of time is difficult, often requiring several medications, and the magnitudes of reductions of risk for CV events and premature mortality for individual patients are relatively small. Therefore, among the many strategies available for lowering CV event risk, BP reduction will not always be the most impactful option. The characteristics of patients most likely to reduce their risk of premature death or disability meaningfully by lowering their BP include those with a) a history of CVA, MI, CHF, CKD, or aneurysm, b) an average systolic BP >150, c) a life expectancy > 5 years, d) a 10-year risk of adverse CV events > 20% after implementing other CV risk reduction strategies, and e) the willingness and ability to maintain effective BP reduction strategies for at least five years.

Several non-pharmacological strategies for lowering systolic BP are safe and effective including:

- Weight loss (if overweight or obese): 5 – 20 mmHg reduction
- DASH or Mediterranean Diet: 8 – 14 mmHg reduction
- Aerobic physical activity 150 min./wk.: 4 – 9 mmHg reduction
- Low sodium diet (< 2.4 gm/day): 2 – 8 mmHg reduction
- Limit alcohol intake to < 2drinks/day if male; <1 drink/day if female: 2 – 4 mmHg reduction
- Aged garlic extract 1200mg twice daily: 8 mmHg

When medications are warranted, it is important to know that while all available antihypertensive medications reduce BP, some lower CV events and all-cause mortality rates more than others. Most effective are thiazide diuretics (MI, CHF), ACE inhibitors (CHF, all-cause mortality), and Ca++channel blockers (CVA). Deserving special mention is ramipril, which, in the HOPE trial, reduced CV events by 40% after controlling for its BP-lowering effect. Ramipril was chosen for that study because of its especially high intracellular ACE inhibition.

Blood Glucose

Blood glucose is another continuous measure with an arbitrary cut-point (126 mg/dl) used to create a disease: diabetes. It is a bit more complicated than blood pressure since higher levels of blood glucose can adversely affect both premature death and disability and current quality of life. Because of pharmaceutical company-sponsored advertising, people fear diabetes and its complications almost as much as they fear cancer. There are a number of different causes and contributing factors, the two most frequent of which are pure beta cell failure (Type 1 diabetes) and insulin resistance plus beta cell insufficiency (Type 2 diabetes; adverse consequences of systemic inflammation).

It is obviously important to know the cause of elevated blood sugar since very low levels of insulin can result in ketoacidosis, coma, and death. Therefore, when prevention of premature death is a goal, all patients with Type 1 diabetes require treatment with insulin or a beta cell transplant. Elevated blood sugar levels of whatever cause can also interfere with the immune response, so careful blood sugar reduction is often warranted during acute illnesses.

Regardless of cause, elevated levels of blood glucose in susceptible individuals can, over 10 – 15 years, cause blindness, kidney failure, nerve damage, and amputations. Risk of those complications depends upon both blood sugar level and life expectancy, since risk rises dramatically after 15 years. For example, microvascular complications are relatively uncommon in patients who develop Type 2 diabetes late in life. If a person develops Type 2 diabetes at age 55, with an A1c of 9% (average blood sugar level of 212 mg/dl) and does nothing to lower it, there is only a 5% chance they will ever go blind or develop kidney failure and a less than 10% chance they will need an amputation. Prevention requires balancing future risk and the potential adverse impacts of hypoglycemia, other medication side effects, cost, inconvenience, and labeling.

Most people with elevated blood glucose caused by type 2 diabetes die or become disabled as a result of heart attacks or strokes. Lowering blood glucose levels has very little impact on those adverse outcomes. While certain medicines used to lower blood sugar levels (e.g., metformin, glucagon-like peptide 1 receptor agonists, and sodium-glucose cotransporter 2 inhibitors) can reduce the risk of cardiovascular events and premature death in patients with cardiovascular disease, the mechanisms appear to have nothing to do with blood sugar reduction.

The most compelling reason to lower blood glucose levels in patients with Type 2 diabetes is to improve their quality of life. Patients with Hgb A1cs above 8% (average blood glucose levels of 205 mg/dl) often have a variety of symptoms that may develop gradually over time and not be reported. When blood sugar levels rise above the renal threshold (usually around 200 mg/dl), glucose spills into the urine, pulling water and salt with it. The result is dehydration, which causes fatigue, weakness, thirst, lightheadedness, dry mouth, dry eyes, dry skin, and constipation. These symptoms resolve when blood sugar levels are reduced, often allowing patients to participate in desired activities.

Interestingly, several sodium-glucose cotransporter 2 inhibitors have recently been developed and are being aggressively advertised. These medicines reduce blood sugar levels by increasing the amount of sugar passing into the urine, which ought to increase dehydration symptoms. In fact, their advertisements admit, "You may experience lightheadedness, fatigue, weakness, and dry mouth. And while it isn't a weight loss medicine, you might lose some weight." However, one ad concludes, "Imagine life with a lower A1c," as if achieving a normal A1c was the goal.

I can see no compelling reason other than established norms to use the label diabetes, and I see even less reason to use the word prediabetes. Prevention of elevated blood glucose levels (i.e., prevention of diabetes) should be viewed within the broader context of reducing systemic inflammation.

Step 8: View Risk Factors as Risk Factors Instead of Diseases

- Health challenges that are important primarily because they can cause premature death or disability are best thought of as risk factors rather than diseases.

Osteopenia

Reduced bone mineral density increases the risk of fractures. It is another example of a continuous measure that has been dichotomized to create the label osteoporosis. Because most fractures also require a fall or other injury, bone mineral density, by itself, is a relatively poor predictor of fractures. Better predictors are age, gender, body mass index, postural instability, and a history of previous fractures. Risk assessment tools (e.g., the Osteoporosis Self-Assessment Tool and FRAX) tend to be evaluated based upon their ability to predict a bone mineral density T-score less than 2.5 rather than their ability to predict fractures.

Weight-bearing physical activity, consuming sufficient quantities of calcium and Vitamin D, exposure to at least 15 minutes of sunlight daily, and avoidance of toxins like cigarette smoke and excessive amounts of alcohol can reduce the rate of bone loss. Lower extremity strengthening and balance exercises like Tai Chi have been shown to reduce the risk of fractures. Older patients with a history of falls can benefit from referral to an occupational and/or physical therapist and an in-home assessment.

Medications that increase bone mineral density by inhibiting bone turnover can reduce the number of vertebral fractures over the next five years by 6% (ARR; from 15% to 9%) and hip fractures by 1% (from 19% to 18%) in individuals who have had a vertebral or hip fracture and by 2% in those at high risk for a vertebral fracture but without a prior fracture. There is no compelling evidence that they prevent hip fractures in patients with no history of a hip fracture. Because they impede remodeling, these medications increase bone fragility and the risk of femoral fractures.

Step 9: Consider Ways to Prevent Chronic Disabling Conditions

- Instead of waiting until damage has been done, consider ways to prevent it from occurring.

Osteoarthritis

Osteoarthritis is still commonly thought of as wear and tear, the inevitable consequence of aging. It isn't. More a syndrome than a single disease, it appears to be the consequence of a wide variety of risk factors that shift the usual balance between cartilaginous breakdown and repair in favor of breakdown. Because osteoarthritis is one of the most common causes of physical disability in older people, it is important for physicians to know what those risk factors are so they can properly advise at-risk patients before symptoms begin to occur. The tables below include a number of established osteoarthritis risk factors. While it may be difficult to convince at-risk patients to implement preventive strategies, it is worth the effort in at least some cases, particularly when the preventive strategies are relatively easy to implement.

Once osteoarthritis has begun to affect quality of life, management should focus on limiting the impact on current and future activities. That might include, in addition to pain management, mitigation of predisposing and aggravating factors and adaptive approaches (e.g., modifying the requirements or activities or using adaptive equipment). It is almost always helpful, therefore, to refer patients with functionally limiting osteoarthritis to physical and/or occupational therapists.

Table 16.3. Genetic and Congenital Factors that Increase Risk for Osteoarthritis

Risk Factor	Proposed Mechanism
Genetic predisposition	Multiple genes identified; multiple mechanisms
Gender (female)	Uncertain mechanism(s)
Ethnicity (European origin)	Association with genetic factors
Overweight/obesity	Uncertain; affects knees and fingers but not hips
Congenital malformations (e.g., excessive joint laxity, malposition)	Repetitive microtrauma

While it may be difficult to convince at-risk patients to implement preventive strategies, it is worth the effort in at least some cases, particularly when the preventive strategies are relatively easy to implement.

Once osteoarthritis has begun to affect quality of life, management should focus on limiting the impact on current and future activities. That might include, in addition to pain management, mitigation of predisposing and aggravating factors and adaptive approaches (e.g., modifying the requirements or activities or using adaptive equipment). It is almost always helpful, therefore, to refer patients with functionally limiting osteoarthritis to physical and/or occupational therapists.

Table 16.4. Occupational and Recreational Risk Factors for Sevelopment of Osteoarthritis

Activity	Occupations
Heavy physical labor	Farming, fisheries, roadwork, weightlifting
High levels of impact and torsion	Football, soccer, basketball, tennis
Kneeling	Mining, floor installation
Stair climbing	Firefighters
Crawling	Plumbing, electricians
Whole-body bending	Stocking (shelves/trucks), construction, nursing aides, housekeeping
Vibration	Pneumatic drilling, truck driving
Repetitive movements	Metal/machinery workers, assembly line, hair cutting / styling

Table 16.5 Toxic and Trauma-Related Risk Factors
for Development of Osteoarthritis

Risk Factor	Proposed Mechanism
Major joint trauma (e,g,, fracture, dislocation)	Deformity or malposition causes ongoing microtrauma
Post-surgical resection (e.g., meniscus surgery)	Deformity or malposition causes ongoing microtrauma
Recurring microtrauma (e.g., occupational, recreational	Ongoing injury overwhelms repair mechanisms
Alcohol	Systemic toxin
Cigarete smoling	Systemic toxin

Table 16.6 Health Challenges that Increase the Risk for
Development of Osteoarthritis

Health Challenge	Proposed Mechanism
Rickets	Deformity or malposition causes ongoing microtrauma plus systemic metabolic effects
Aseptic osteonecrosis	Deformity or malposition causing ongoing microtrauma plus systemic metabolic effects
Hemochromatosis	Iron deposition in cartilage contributing to breakdown and/or impeding repair
Hyperuricemia	Uric acid deposition in cartilage contributing to breakdown and/or impeding repair
Hyperparathyroidism	Calcium deposition in cartilage contributing to breakdown and/or impeding repair

Chondrocalcinosis	Calcium deposition in cartilage contributes to breakdown and/or impedes repair
Acromegaly	Bone and cartilage enlargement causing deformity and micro-trauma
Onchronosis	Homogentisic acid deposition in cartilage contributes to break-down and impedes repair

Step 10: Learn to Ask the Should Question

- In addition to the question, "Can this condition be treated," learn to ask, "Should it be treated?" and, if so, "When?" Of course, the answers to those questions will depend upon the answer to the why question. What is the goal?
- Upper Respiratory Tract Infections
- Acute, self-limited health challenges are primarily relevant to quality of life and personal growth and development until and unless serious complications occur. Perhaps the best example is upper respiratory infections.
- We now have sufficient evidence to make recommendations about treatment of upper respiratory infections (URIs), including acute rhinitis, pharyngitis, otitis media, sinusitis, and laryngitis, as well as self-limited lower respiratory infections (LRIs), including tracheitis and bronchitis, in patients with otherwise normal respiratory tracts and immune systems. Since URIs rarely cause premature death, the relevant goals of care for most patients are improving current quality of life and promoting personal growth and development (knowledge and resilience). It is therefore important to know how the symptoms are affecting the patient's daily life. Often all that is needed is reassurance and perhaps a note for school or

work. It is also important to assess the patient's understanding of their illness.

- Aside from streptococcal and gonococcal pharyngitis, differentiating between viral and bacterial etiologies is unimportant since nearly all episodes, regardless of organism, resolve on their own without complications. While antibiotics may shorten the duration of some symptoms (e.g., the pain associated with acute otitis media) by 12-24 hours, their short- and long-term adverse effects generally outweigh those minor benefits.

- Rather than worrying about whether the pathogen can be killed with antibiotics, the more important concern is which patients are likely to develop prolonged or complicated infections. At present, the only reliable ways to do that are to consider risk factors and past history and/or to wait five to seven days to see whether the symptoms are improving or getting worse. An added benefit of a wait-and-see approach is that the immune system has a chance to respond and become better able to handle the next infection. One proven way to sell this approach to skeptical patients is to provide a delayed prescription to be filled after a specified number of days if the symptoms are worsening.

- Fortunately, most patients understand the importance of avoiding antibiotics when possible. However, if patients insist on antibiotic treatment, arguing is generally a waste of time. It is more helpful to use that time to discuss how to keep from spreading the current infection, how to prevent future infections, and what to do when they occur. As for over-the-counter cold remedies, most of which are designed to prevent the body from ridding itself of the invading organisms, the evidence of benefit is weak at best and usually not worth the cost or adverse effects but also not worth arguing about.

Step 11: Learn to Use Medications Cautiously

- Be extremely cautious about prescribing medications of any kind.

Rules for Prescribing and Managing Medications

1. You always overestimate the value and underestimate the harms caused by medications, even if you consider this rule.

2. Never prescribe a medication unless absolutely necessary. If intervention is required, always consider non-pharmacologic strategies first (e.g., ice, heat, exercise).

3. Try to limit the number of systemically active medications to five or less. If you are tempted to start a sixth medication, see if you can stop a current one. Any benefit of additional medications is likely to be offset by side effects, interactions, and administration errors.

4. For EVERY new symptom, think FIRST about the possibility that it could be a medication side effect.

5. Require patients to bring all of their regular medications, both prescription and non-prescription, with them to every clinic visit. Make sure this message is reinforced in as many different ways as possible. Update the patient's medication list at every visit.

6. Ask patients to contact you if possible before adding any new prescription medication to their regimen. Make sure your patients know that you want to be involved in all medication decisions.

7. On admission to the hospital, before putting patients on the medications they are supposed to be taking, try to determine if they have actually been taking the medications as prescribed.

8. Start at the lowest possible dose and increase the dose slowly enough to detect adverse effects before they are severe. View the administration of every new medicine as a chemical experiment in which all of the possible effects are not known.

9. When discontinuing a medication, consider tapering it rather than stopping it cold turkey, especially when the patient has been on it for a long time.

10. Try really hard not to change a patient's medications at the first visit. Patients often come to a new physician because they have a

suspicion that something bad is going to happen. If you change a medicine and something bad happens, both you and the patient are going to think you caused it.

Step 12: Plan for Adjustments

- Nearly all plans require adjustments based upon unforeseen obstacles and challenges. Most plans fail initially. Learn to view the causes of these failures as bits of additional information rather than as non-adherence. Schedule follow-up phone calls on the assumption that adjustments will need to be made. Adjustments can involve reconsideration of goals, objectives, and/or strategies. ***

Appendix A: Risk Factors

This is the list of risk factors and risk reduction strategies used for the health risk appraisal algorithm developed by Dr. Nagykaldi. It takes between 20–30 minutes for most patients to complete on a computer.

General

How far did you go in school?
☐ Less than a high-school diploma ☐ High-school graduate or GED ☐ Some college, no degree ☐ Associate degree ☐ Bachelor's degree ☐ Master's degree ☐ Professional degree ☐ Doctoral degree

What is your marital status?
☐ Married ☐ Widowed ☐ Single ☐ Separated or Divorced

Gender Assigned at Birth
☐ Male ☐ Female

How do you describe yourself?
☐ Male ☐ Female ☐ Trans-gender-male ☐ Trans-gender-Female ☐ Other

What is your sexual orientation?
☐ Heterosexual (straight) ☐ Gay ☐ Lesbian ☐ Bisexual ☐ Other

What is your primary race?
☐ White ☐ African American ☐ American Indian ☐ Asian/Pacific Islander ☐ Other

What is your ethnicity?
☐ Hispanic/Latino ☐ Ashkenazi Jewish ☐ Unknown

What is the location of your place of residence?
☐ Urban ☐ Suburban ☐ Rural

How does your household income compare to the local median household income?
☐ Less than half of median ☐ Below median ☐ About median ☐ Above median ☐ Over twice the median

What is your employment status?
☐ Employed ☐ Unemployed ☐ Looking for a job ☐ Student ☐ Homemaker ☐ Retired ☐ Disabled

Diet, Physical Activity, Alcohol, and Tobacco

How many servings of the following food groups do you eat on a typical day (e.g., Choose yesterday or today if either was fairly typical)?

Dairy (one serving = 1 cup)

☐ 0 ☐ 1 ☐ 2 ☐ 3 ☐ 4 ☐ 5+

Grains (one serving = 1 cup)

☐ 0 ☐ 1 ☐ 2 ☐ 3 ☐ 4 ☐ 5+

Meat (one serving = deck of cards size)

☐ 0 ☐ 1 ☐ 2 ☐ 3 ☐ 4 ☐ 5+

Fruits (one serving = medium apple size)

☐ 0 ☐ 1 ☐ 2 ☐ 3 ☐ 4 ☐ 5+

Vegetables (one serving = half cup size)

☐ 0 ☐ 1 ☐ 2 ☐ 3 ☐ 4 ☐ 5+

Do you regularly eat foods high in cholesterol, saturated fat or trans-fat (e.g. eggs, butter, bacon or fatty meat, shortening, and hard margarine)?

☐ Yes ☐ No

Do you eat more than 3 servings of red or processed meat during a typical WEEK (1 serving size is about a deck of cards of red meat, sausage, hamburger, or liver)

☐ Yes ☐ No

Do you regularly eat food that was prepared by frying, broiling, or grilling at high temperatures?

☐ Yes ☐ No

How many servings of carbs do you think you might eat on a typical day (1 serving can be found in 1 slice of bread, 4-6 crackers, 1 small fresh fruit, 1 small potato, half cup of cooked beans, peas, or corn, half cup of fruit juice)?

☐ <8 ☐ 9 ☐ 10 ☐ 11 ☐ 12 ☐ 13 ☐ 14 ☐ 15 ☐ 16+

Have you made an effort to reduce your intake of sodium (table salt)?

☐ Yes ☐ No

How would you describe your level of physical activity (averaged over a typical week)?

☐ Sedentary (minimal activity)   ☐ Insufficiently active (occasional, moderate activity)   ☐

Stress, Sleep, and Safety

Can you describe your life as unusually stressful?

☐ Yes ☐ No

How many major life events have you experienced recently (e.g. death of a loved one, divorce, or job loss) that you feel are difficult to cope with?

☐ 0 ☐ 1 ☐ 2 ☐ 3+

How many hours of sleep do you usually get on a typical day?

☐ <6 ☐ 6-7 ☐ 7-8 ☐ 8-9 ☐ >9

Do you have a physical impairment or disability that interferes with your daily living (limits what you can do)?

☐ Yes ☐ No

Do you live in a neighborhood with a high violent crime rate?

☐ Yes ☐ No

Do you live with a violent or abusive person?

☐ Yes ☐ No

Past Health Challenges

Do you have a personal history of any of the following conditions?

Hypertension (high blood pressure)

☐ No ☐ Treated ☐ Untreated

Metabolic syndrome

☐ No ☐ Yes

Diabetes / pre-diabetes

☐ No ☐ Type I ☐ Type II ☐ Prediabetes

Rheumatoid arthritis

☐ No ☐ Yes

Clinical depression

☐ No ☐ Yes

Stroke

☐ No ☐ Yes

Heart attack or transient ischemic attack (TIA)

☐ No ☐ Yes

Congestive heart failure (CHF)

☐ No ☐ Yes

Atrial fibrillation

☐ No ☐ Yes

Other heart or blood vessel problems (including atherosclerosis, varicose veins, aneurysm, and blood vessel inflammation)

☐ No ☐ Yes

Chronic obstructive pulmonary disease (COPD) (e.g., chronic bronchitis or emphysema)

☐ No ☐ Stage 0 ☐ Stage I ☐ Stage II ☐ Stage III ☐ Stage IV

Asthma

☐ No ☐ Yes, but it does not disrupt my life (under control) ☐ Yes, and it disrupts my life (not

Alzheimer's disease

☐ No ☐ Yes

Parkinson's disease

☐ No ☐ Yes

Systemic lupus erythematosus (SLE)

☐ No ☐ Yes

Chronic kidney disease

☐ No ☐ Stage I ☐ Stage II ☐ Stage III ☐ Stage IV ☐ Stage V (End-Stage)

Chronic liver disease

☐ No ☐ Alcoholic Type ☐ Hepatitis B or C Type ☐ Primary biliary cirrhosis Type

Chronic hepatitis B or C

☐ No ☐ Yes

Microalbuminuria

☐ No ☐ Yes

Peripheral artery disease

☐ No ☐ Yes

Impaired glucose tolerance

☐ No ☐ Yes

Cancer (any type) or your doctor told you that you have cancer genes

☐ No ☐ Yes

Lung cancer

☐ No ☐ Stage I ☐ Stage II ☐ Stage IIIA ☐ Stage IIIB ☐ Stage IV ☐ Limited small cell ☐ Advanced small cell

Bladder cancer

☐ No ☐ Stage T-0 ☐ Stage T-is/T-a ☐ Stage T1 ☐ Stage T2a/T2b ☐ Stage T3 ☐ Stage T4a ☐ Stage T4b

Kidney cancer

☐ No ☐ Stage I ☐ Stage II ☐ Stage III ☐ Stage IV

Pancreatic cancer

☐ No ☐ Localized stage ☐ Regional stage ☐ Distant stage

Melanoma skin cancer

☐ No ☐ Localized stage ☐ Regional stage ☐ Distant stage

Non-melanoma skin cancer (squamous cell carcinoma)

☐ No ☐ Early stage ☐ Advanced stage ☐ Basal cell carcinoma

Prostate cancer

☐ No ☐ Stage I ☐ Stage II ☐ Stage III ☐ Stage IV

Colorectal cancer

☐ No ☐ Stage I ☐ Stage IIA ☐ Stage IIB ☐ Stage IIIA ☐ Stage IIIB ☐ Stage IIIC ☐ Stage IV

Sleep apnea

☐ No ☐ Yes

Head injury after 50 years of age

☐ No ☐ Yes

Glomerulonephritis (a type of inflamed kidneys)

☐ No ☐ Yes

Recent complication of a urinary tract infection (e.g. kidney infection)

☐ No ☐ Yes

Kidney or bladder stones

☐ No ☐ Yes

Recent major injury (any type)

☐ No ☐ Yes

Debilitating physical illnesses

☐ No ☐ Yes

Biliary obstruction (gall duct closure)

☐ No ☐ Yes

Hemochromatosis

☐ No ☐ Yes

Family Health Challenges

Do you have a FAMILY history of the following conditions?
(First degree relatives are: parent, sibling, and child; second degree relatives are: grandparent, grandchild, uncle, aunt, nephew, niece, and half-sibling.)

Cardiovascular disease and/or death due to cardiovascular disease before age 75 in first degree relative
☐ No ☐ Father ☐ Mother ☐ Both ☐ Not sure

Lung cancer in first degree relative
☐ No ☐ Relative diagnosed before age 60 ☐ Relative diagnosed after age 60 ☐ Not sure

Breast cancer in first or second degree relative
☐ No ☐ Yes ☐ Yes, relative diagnosed before age 50 ☐ Yes, male relative with breast cancer ☐ Not sure

Pancreatic cancer in first degree relative
☐ No ☐ Yes ☐ Not sure

Prostate cancer in first degree relative
☐ No ☐ Father only ☐ Brother only ☐ Other first degree relative ☐ Two or more relatives ☐ Not sure

Colorectal cancer in first degree relative
☐ No ☐ One relative ☐ Two or more relatives ☐ Not sure

Ovarian cancer in first or second degree relative
☐ No ☐ One relative ☐ Two or more relatives ☐ Not sure

Cervical cancer in first degree relative
☐ No ☐ Yes ☐ Not sure

Stroke in first degree relative
☐ No ☐ Yes ☐ Not sure

Diabetes in first degree relative
☐ No ☐ One relative ☐ Two or more relatives ☐ Not sure

Alzheimer's disease in first degree relative
☐ No ☐ One parent or sibling ☐ Both parents or siblings ☐ Not sure

Chronic kidney disease in first degree relative
☐ No ☐ Yes ☐ Not sure

Suicide in first degree relative
☐ No ☐ Yes ☐ Not sure

Hypertension (high blood pressure) in first degree relative

☐ No ☐ Mother ☐ Father ☐ Both ☐ Not sure

Parkinson's disease in first or second degree relative

☐ No ☐ Diagnosed before age 70 ☐ Diagnosed after age 70 ☐ Not sure

Melanoma skin cancer in first degree relative

☐ No ☐ Yes ☐ Not sure

Have you been hospitalized or admitted to a nursing home in the last 6 months?

☐ Yes ☐ No

Did you have a major surgery in the last year?

☐ Yes ☐ No

How many times did you visit a doctor's office in the last year?

☐ 0 ☐ 1 ☐ 2 ☐ 3 ☐ 4 ☐ 5 ☐ 6 ☐ 7 ☐ 8 ☐ 9 ☐ 10+

How many times did you go to the Emergency Room (ER) in the last year?

☐ 0 ☐ 1 ☐ 2 ☐ 3 ☐ 4 ☐ 5 ☐ 6 ☐ 7 ☐ 8 ☐ 9 ☐ 10+

Current Allergies and Immunological Deficiencies

Do you currently have a compromised or weakened immune system?

☐ Yes ☐ No

Immunosuppression (e.g., because of an organ transplant or chronic inflammatory condition like psoriasis, rheumatoid arthritis, lupus, or inflammatory bowel disease)

☐ No ☐ Yes

Are you allergic to eggs?

☐ Yes ☐ No

Have you ever received Gamma-globulin or transfusion?

☐ Yes ☐ No

Did you have varicella (chickenpox)?

☐ Yes ☐ No

Have you ever had Guillain-Barre syndrome?

☐ Yes ☐ No

Have you had a colectomy (removal of a part of the large intestine)?

☐ Yes ☐ No

Have you been diagnosed with HIV/AIDS?

☐ Yes ☐ No

Mental Health Challenges

Do you live with individuals who have a history of mental problems such as depression, mood disorder, schizophrenia, and anxiety disorder?

Yes   No

Over the last 2 weeks, how often have you been bothered by any of the following problems?

Little interest or pleasure in doing things

Not at all   Several days   More than half the days   Nearly every day

Feeling down, depressed, or hopeless

Not at all   Several days   More than half the days   Nearly every day

Have you been told by a doctor that you have clinical depression which may require treatment?

☐ Yes ☐ No

How would you rate your mental activity (thinking, learning, reasoning) in general?

☐ Low ☐ Average ☐ High

Have you ever attempted suicide?

☐ Yes, and I still have nightmares   ☐ Yes, but I do not have nightmares   ☐ No

Do you have a history of significant physiological trauma or abuse?

☐ Yes ☐ No

Did you experience a traumatic event in your life that still has a strong effect on you?

☐ Yes ☐ No

Risk Reduction Strategies

Do you usually wear sunscreen when you spend extended time outside during the summer?

☐ Yes ☐ No

Do you always buckle your seatbelt?

☐ Yes ☐ No

How many miles do you usually travel by car in a year (approximate)?

Do you use your cell phone to talk or text while driving?

☐ Yes ☐ No ☐ I do not drive

Do you always wear a helmet when bicycling, skating, boarding, etc?

☐ I do not bike, skate, or board   ☐ Yes I always wear a helmet   ☐ I do not always wear a helmet

Do you have a working smoke alarm in your home?

☐ Yes ☐ No

Did you fall inside or outside of your home recently that resulted in an injury?

☐ Yes ☐ No

Do you often ride a motorcycle?

☐ Yes, with a helmet ☐ Without helmet ☐ No

Do you have easy access to weapons or own weapons?

☐ Yes, and I live alone ☐ Yes, and I live with others ☐ No

Please indicate which preventive services you receive currently or received in the period shown:

Hearing testing

☐ Yes ☐ Never ☐ Does not apply Approx. date (if known):

Vision screening

☐ Yes, periodically ☐ No ☐ Does not apply Approx. date (if known):

I am taking baby aspirin on a regular basis

☐ Yes ☐ No

I am taking an ACE inhibitor (e.g. lisinopril, captopril) or angiotensin receptor blocker / ARB medication (e.g. Cozaar, Hyzaar, Atacand, Avapro) for my blood pressure or heart problem

☐ Yes ☐ No

I am on a cholesterol lowering medication (e.g. Lipitor, Zocor, Crestor)

☐ Yes ☐ No

My cholesterol was checked in the last

☐ Year ☐ 2 years ☐ 5 years ☐ Not in 5 years Approx. date (if known):

I am on insulin

☐ Yes ☐ No

I had colorectal cancer screening

☐ Colonoscopy in last 10 years ☐ Sigmoidoscopy in last 5 years ☐ Stool cards in last year ☐ No ☐ Does not apply Approx. date (if known):

I received a pneumonia shot (pneumococcal vaccine)

☐ Yes ☐ Never ☐ Does not apply Approx. date (if known):

I got a flu shot during the most recent flu season

☐ Yes ☐ No ☐ Does not apply Approx. date (if known):

I can rate my overall health in the last month as (do not count an occasional infection, e.g. the fl

☐ Very good ☐ Good ☐ Average ☐ Bad ☐ Very bad

I can rate my satisfaction with my life (1 - not at all satisfied >> 10 - extremely satisfied):

☐ 1 ☐ 2 ☐ 3 ☐ 4 ☐ 5 ☐ 6 ☐ 7 ☐ 8 ☐ 9 ☐ 10

Appendix B: Advance Directives

This is the set of questions we asked every patient in our geriatric clinic every year as part of a comprehensive questionnaire).

Since we know that we will all die someday, it is a good idea to think about your values and preferences for how you would like it to happen. **Please complete the following questionnaire. We encourage you to discuss your answers with loved ones and others who might have to make decisions for you at the end of your life.**

VALUES HISTORY: The following questions will help us a great deal in taking care of your medical needs. IT IS NOT A LEGAL DOCUMENT. It is **not** a **living will**. Your answers help us understand your values and preferences.

I want to live as long as I can. If necessary, I want all medical interventions used to help me live longer. My quality of life is not as important as living as long as I can.

I want to keep a good quality of life. I do not want medical interventions used to make me live longer. My quality of life matters a great deal to me.

Many different values help each of us define the quality of life we would like to live. Please review the following list, and feel free to add any statements that you want. **Then check the THREE that are the most important to you.**

I want to maintain my capacity to think clearly.

I want to feel safe and secure.

I want to avoid unnecessary pain and suffering.

I want to be treated with respect.

I want to be treated with dignity when I can no longer speak for myself.

I do not want to be an unnecessary burden on my family.

I want to maintain a good relationship with my family.

I want to be able to be with loved ones before I die.

I want to be able to make my own decisions.

I want to experience a comfortable dying process.

I want to leave good memories of myself to my loved ones.

I want to be treated in accord with my religious beliefs and traditions.

I want respect shown for my body after I die.

I want to help others by making a contribution to medical education and research.

Other important values:

_____

_____

_____

Your answers to the following questions will help us a great deal in taking care of your medical needs. Please answer them to the best of your ability. It is not a legal document. It is NOT a living will.

1. Do you want to receive cardiopulmonary resuscitation (CPR) if your heart should stop beating? (today, in your current state of health)   Yes   No   Don't know

2. Do you want to be put on a respirator (breathing machine) temporarily if your lungs should fail? (today, in your current state of health)   Yes   No   Don't know

NOTE: Use of a respirator requires a tube to be put through your nose or mouth into your lungs and connected to a breathing machine.

3. If you lose consciousness or become confused and there is not enough time to reach your doctor, do you want someone to take you to an emergency room? (today, in your current state of health)   Yes   No   Don't know

4. Do you have a **living will**? (Advance Directive for Health Care)   Yes   No   Don't know

5. Do you have a durable **power of attorney**?   Yes   No   Don't know

   Name: _____

   Address: _____ Phone: _____

6. Has a guardian been appointed for you?   Yes   No   Don't know

   Name:

   Address: _____ Phone: _____

7. Who will help you make decisions about your medical care if you cannot and if you have no durable power of attorney or guardian?

   Name: _____

   Address: _____ Phone

   _____

   Name: _____

   Address _____ Phone

8. When you die, do you want to donate your organs for transplantation?   Yes   No   Don't know

9. Would you allow an autopsy upon your death? (If it would help your family or your doctors.)   Yes   No   Don't know   v

10. What activities are REALLY important to you (without which life would lose much of its meaning)?

11   Would any of the following conditions, if permanent, be **WORSE THAN DEATH?**

___living in a nursing home

___unable to live by myself

___unable to make decisions for myself

too confused to recognize family members

an incurable terminal illness associated with severe pain

___a permanent vegetative state (heart and lungs alive but no brain activity)

___other _____

12.   Who besides those involved in your health care would you let have information about your medical condition?

Name_____

Name_____

13.   Have you communicated with family
members the location of important
documents such as deeds,
titles, insurance policies,
safety deposit box, living will and regular will?

Yes   No   Donít know

Appendix C: Patient Education

These are examples of the kinds of patient education materials that you will want to create.

Goal-Oriented Health Care

Much of the medical care you have received in the past has focused on solving problems. The assumption is that correcting abnormalities will result in a longer and more enjoyable life. However, it is an indirect approach that can be somewhat mechanical and impersonal and can too often result in unnecessary tests and treatments.

We prefer a more direct and positive approach. We try to help you develop a plan of care based upon your personal values and your health-related goals and priorities. Focusing directly on your goals and priorities helps assure that tests and treatments will be relevant.

We assume that you want to live as long as possible up to the point when life is no longer worth living, and that you want to be able to do the things that you enjoy and find meaningful. We hope you also want to become stronger and more adaptable and resilient, and at the end of your life, we would like for you to have a good death. While we have those goals in common, each of us has a unique set of risk factors, resources and strengths, values, hopes, preferences, priorities.

Our intention is to create a long-term relationship with you and, if possible, with your family in which we can work together to help you achieve your goals in the ways that you define them. That will require a somewhat greater investment on both of our parts than what you may have experienced with your previous health care providers.

As soon as possible we would like to schedule a new patient evaluation and wellness visit. Prior to that visit, we are assigning some homework. Please complete the attached questionnaire to the best of your ability. Also, complete and sign Request for Medical Records forms for each medical practice in which you have been seen more than twice or had laboratory or other tests (X-rays, colonoscopies, etc.) done within the last 5 years, and each hospital in which you were either seen in the Emergency Department or admitted overnight during that same time period. Bring the completed questionnaire and signed forms to your visit along with all of the medications and supplements you take on a regular basis in a plastic bag or other suitable container.

At every visit, be prepared to discuss the activities you are having trouble with, those you wish you could do more of, and those that are particularly important to you.

Physical Activity

A minimum amount of physical activity is needed to make your body work properly. You won't feel as good or live as long if you don't get at least 90 to 150 minutes of moderate physical activity per week. Moderate physical activity is activity that raises your heart and breathing rate to a level where you can still talk but you can't sing. It doesn't count unless you do it for at least 10 minutes at a time. An ideal routine then would involve about 30 minutes 3 to 5 times a week.

A deficiency of physical activity can cause or contribute to nearly every possible symptom from trouble thinking, to trouble sleeping to joint pain, to constipation. It is like a vitamin deficiency but worse, since it affects every function in the body. Long-term physical activity deficiency results in premature aging and a reduced life expectancy.

When deciding how to get your weekly requirement of physical activity, there are several things you should consider.

1. Since much of the additional life you will gain from physical activity will be spent doing physical activity, pick something you enjoy. If you don't enjoy any kind of physical activity, remember it isn't optional; pick something you can tolerate. Remember that 150 minutes per week is only 1.4% of your week. You can do it!

2. If possible, engage in your chosen activity with someone else who

can help keep you motivated when you are tired, the weather is poor, life becomes more stressful, etc.

3. If you have been inactive for more than a few weeks, start slowly and build up gradually with both the duration and intensity of the activity.

4. If you have arthritis or some other condition that makes physical activity difficult or painful, ask us for advice and possibly a referral to a physical therapist.

Heart Attacks and Angina

The coronary arteries are small blood vessels that supply the heart muscle with oxygen and nutrition. When the insides of the coronary arteries are injured by elevated pressure, inflammation from obesity and inactivity, or exposure to chemicals from smoking, cholesterol-filled plaques can form.

If a plaque breaks open, a clot may develop, blocking the flow of blood. If flow is blocked for more than a few hours, the heart muscle dies. That is a heart attack. Heart attacks can cause weakening of the heart muscle and serious problems with the heart's rhythm.

The usual symptoms of a heart attack are pressure, tightness, and pain in the left or central part of the chest that may radiate to the left arm and neck. It can be associated with sweating, nausea, shortness of breath, weakness, and lightheadedness.

If you think you may be having a heart attack, call for an ambulance to take you to the nearest hospital immediately. It is possible to reopen the blocked artery, preventing permanent damage.

You can estimate your risk of having a heart attack using risk calculators like ASCVD () or Framingham (). Tests like the cardiac calcium scan and the CRP blood test don't usually add very much to these estimates.

You can reduce your heart attack risk by reducing further damage and preventing clots. You can: 1) stop smoking and avoid exposure to second-hand smoke; 2) engage in moderate physical activity at least 90 minutes per week; 3) reduce your average systolic blood pressure (top number) to less than 140; 4) take a statin medicine at the highest dose you can tolerate or enough to lower your LDL cholesterol ("bad cholesterol") level to less than 100 mg/dl; 5) reduce your weight to achieve a body mass index (BMI) of 26 or less; and/or 6) take low-dose aspirin (81mg daily) if you are at particularly high risk.

If a number of plaques form over a period of time, and they don't break open, they can become hardened with calcium and scar tissue and can eventually block the flow of blood. Because it happens gradually, the body can usually create new blood vessels around the blockages. However, when the flow of blood is insufficient, chest pain can result. That pain, which is called angina, is similar to the pain of a heart attack but much less severe, and it doesn't last very long. It is brought on by physical activity, emotional distress, exposure to heat or cold, or a meal and is relieved promptly by resting.

If you think you may be having angina, see your primary care physician, but not as an emergency. If the symptom isn't new and isn't changing, you can safely wait for the next available appointment. Go directly to the emergency room if the pain is new or if it is occurring much more often with less exertion or stress and lasting longer than 5 minutes despite resting.

Angina can be reduced with medicines that protect the heart from stress and by procedures that either reopen (angioplasty with stenting) the blocked arteries or bypass them with grafts. Those procedures do not, however, prevent heart attacks.

Appendix D: Clinical Decision Support
or Prevention

These are examples of online resources that are helpful when practicing goal-directed care.

Estimating Life Expectancy

General Life Expectancy Calculators
- *https://www.blueprintincome.com/tools/life-expectancy-calculator-how-long-will-i-live/*
- *https://eprognosis.ucsf.edu/lee.php*
- *https://www.projectbiglife.ca/life-expectancy-calculator*

By Location of Home
- *https://qz.com/1462111/map-what-story-does-your-neighborhoods-life-expectancy-tell/*

For Patients with Cancer (by organ, cell type, stage, and grade)
- *https://cancersurvivalrates.com/calculator.html?sex=M&age=65&stage=2&grade=moderately&diagnosed=0&histologyco=adenocarcinoma&type=colon&years=5&role=doctor*

Cardiovascular Risk Calculators (Mayo)
- *https://shareddecisions.mayoclinic.org/decision-aid-information/decision-aids-for-chronic-disease/cardiovascular-prevention/*
- *https://www.rpr.lib.ok.us/resource/prediction-individual-life-years-gained-without-cardiovascular-events-lipid-blood-pressure*
- *http://hf-risk-calculator.surge.sh/*

10-Year Mortality Calculator
- *https://eprognosis.ucsf.edu/calculators/#/*
    Multiple Risk Calculators (Cleveland Clinic)
- *https://riskcalc.org/*

Decision Aids

Decision Aids by Health Topic
https://decisionaid.ohri.ca/AZlist.html

Decision Aids for Colon and Breast Cancer screening, and LVADs and ICDs for Advanced Heart Failure
https://eprognosis.ucsf.edu/decision_aids.php

Mayo Shared Decision-Making Resource Center
https://shareddecisions.mayoclinic.org/decision-aid-information/decision-aids-for-chronic-disease/

Appendix E: Clinical Care Pathways

These are examples of the care pathways discussed in Chapters 12 and 16.

Smoking Cessation

Brief History

_____

_____

_____

Reason Patient Wants to Quit (Goal)

_____

Practice Contacts

Person: _____

    Method: phone, e-mail, text message, in-office, in-home____

    Contact Information: _____

Access Issues:

    Transportation: _____ Mobility: ____ Sensory: ____

    Language: _____ Literacy: _____

    Other: _____

Evaluation:

    Heaviness of Smoking Index

Strategies:

    Formal Support:

        Quit Line: 1-800-784-8669 (1-800-QUITNOW)

        Tobacco cessation program (local)

        Becomeanex.org (web-based support program)

        Smokefree.gov (text messaging program)

        Acupuncture

        Other: _____

Medication: nicotine replacement, Chantix, bupropion_____
Informal Support (e.g., spouse, co-worker) _____
Behavioral Strategies: Activities, relationships, distractions,
rewards_____

_____

Other Strategies:

_____

_____

Follow-up:

Quit Date: _____

Planned contact dates:

_____

_____

_____

Unplanned Contacts: phone call, office visit (when, how):

_____

_____

Trouble Sleeping

Brief History

_____

_____

_____

Reason Patient Wants to Improve Sleep (Goal)

_____

Practice Contacts

Person:

Method: phone, e-mail, text message, in-office, in-home

_____

Contact Information: _____

Access Issues:

Transportation: ____ Mobility: _____ Sensory: _____

Language: ____ Literacy: _____ Other: ____

Evaluation:

    Questionnaires:

        Children: PSQ, _____

        Adolescents: SII, _____

        Adults: STOP, Epworth, _____

    Sleep Studies:

   Home, Sleep Lab   Company/Lab/Consultant: _____

Strategies:

    Stop or reduce current medications (stimulants,
        sedatives), diet (caffeine), and alcohol

    Sleep Hygiene Instructions/Handout

    Cognitive Behavioral Therapy: formal, self-administered
        Therapist: _____

    Sleep Consultant: _____

    PAP: CPAP, BiPAP, VPAP

    Meds and Supplements: melatonin, doxepin, Ambien

    _____

    Other Strategies:

    _____

Follow-up:

    Planned contact dates:

    _____

    _____

    _____

    Unplanned Contacts: phone call, office visit:

    _____

Excessive Use of Alcohol

Brief History

_____

_____

_____

Reason Patient Wants to Reduce Alcohol Consumption (Goal)

_____

Practice Contacts

Person:

Method: phone, e-mail, text message, in-office, in-home

Contact Information: _____

Access Issues:

Transportation: _____ Mobility: _____ Sensory: _____

Language: _____ Literacy: _____ Other: _____

Evaluation:

Questionnaire: AUDIT

Strategies:

Soft handoff to AA

Alcohol abuse counseling

Medication-Assisted Therapy: Antabuse, naltrexone,

Campral

_____

Other Strategies: _____

Follow-up:

Planned contact dates:

_____

_____

_____

Unplanned Contacts: phone call, office visit,:

_____

Alcohol Misuse

- Validated alcohol use questionnaires (e.g., AUDIT, ASSIST, CAGE, DAST-10)
- Medication assisted therapy
- Soft handoff to alcohol abuse counselor or AA sponsor
- Facilitated referral for inpatient therapy

Pathways for immunizations would depend upon practice size, age distribution, and availability of outside resources.

Childhood Immunizations

Depending upon the number of children in the practice and the availability of public and community resources, the practice might develop an immunization station where parents could bring children in any time for their immunizations in addition to well child care visits or all childhood immunizations could be referred to the health department.

Adult Immunizations

In many circumstances, the best way to handle adult immunizations may be to refer patients to their pharmacy. Alternatively, they could be given in conjunction with wellness visits.

Pathways for screening might include the following features.

Cancer Screening

Screening pathways should always include an eligibility algorithm. Depending upon the number of eligible patients, a practice might reserve a block of appointments in the mammography and colonoscopy practices so that appointments could be directly scheduled. CT scanning for lung cancer and Ultrasound scanning for abdominal aortic aneurysm could be built into the smoking cessation pathway and/or be included in the cancer screening pathway.

Pathways for some common tertiary preventive strategies like blood pressure, cholesterol, or blood sugar reduction might include the following components.

Blood Pressure Reduction

Once a target blood pressure level has been established for an individual patient, a standard algorithm could be implemented beginning with evaluation, then lifestyle change options, then a set of medication progressions based upon co-existing risk factors such as renal or hepatic failure.

Citations

This is a list of citations for articles and books specifically mentioned in each section. Articles mentioned more than once, like my 1991 Family Medicine article and the article by Bortz on disuse and aging, are listed in the section in which they are first mentioned. Under the Forward section, I have also listed some articles, one book chapter, and my first book, which are referred to generally but not specifically. Otherwise, I have not attempted to reference most of the statements made in the book.

Preface

Mold JW, Blake GH, and Becker LA. (1991) Goal-oriented medical care. *Family Medicine*, 23:46-51.

Mold JW, Hamm R., & Jafri B. (2000) The effect of labeling on perceived ability to recover from acute illnesses and injuries. *The Journal of Family Practice*, 49(5):437-440.

Mold JW. (2017) Goal-directed health care: Redefining health and health care in the era of value-based care. *Cureus*, 9(2): e1043. *http://www.cureus.com/articles/5935-goal-directed-health-care-redefining-health-and-health-care-in-the-era-of-value-based-care?utm_medium=email&utm_source=transaction.*

Kuhn TS. (2012) *The Structure of Scientific Revolutions* (4th ed.), University of Chicago Press, Chicago, IL.

Introduction

Mold JW. (1995) An alternative conceptualization of health and health care: Its implications for geriatrics and gerontology. *Educational Gerontology*, 21:85-101.

Mold JW, and McCarthy L. (1995) Pearls from geriatrics, or a long line at the bathroom. *The Journal of Family Practice*: 41(1):22-23.

Mold JW, and Knapp KR. (1996) Interdisciplinary Teamwork. In Schmele, June A. (Ed.), *Quality Management in Nursing and Health Care* (pp. 125-137). Delmar Publishing, Inc., Albany, NY.

Zubialde JP, Mold JW. (2001) Relational value: Bridging the worldview gap between patients and health systems. *Family Medicine*, 33(5):393-397.

Mold JW, Hamm R, and Scheid D. (2003) Evidence-based medicine meets goal-directed health care. *Family Medicine*, 35(5):360-364.

Zubialde J, and Mold JW. (2009) Outcomes that matter in chronic illness: An approach informed by self-determination and adult-learning theory. *Families, Systems, & Health*, 27(3): 193-200.

Mold JW. (2017) *Achieving Your Personal Health Goals: A Patient's Guide.* Full Court Press, Chapel Hill, NC.

Reuben DB. and Tinetti ME. (2012) Goal-Oriented Patient Care – An Alternative Outcomes Paradigm. *NEJM*, 366(9): 777- 779.

De Maeseneer J. James W. Mold and colleagues on the shift to goal-oriented medical care. In *Family Medicine: The Classic Papers* (Michael Kidd, Iona Heath, and Amanda Howe, Eds.)

Tanenbaum SJ. (2015) What is Patient-Centered Care? A Typology of Models and Missions. *Health Care Anal*, 23(3):272-287.

Miles A, and Mezzich J. (2015) The care of the patient and the soul of the clinic: person centered medicine as an emergent model. *Health Care Analysis*, 23: 272-287.

Eklund JH, Holmström IK, Ķumlin T, Kaminsky E, Skoglund K, et al. (2019) Same same or different? A review of reviews of person-centered and patient-centered care. *Patient Education and Counseling,* 102(1): 3-11

Gladwell M. (1976) *The Tipping Point: How Little Things Can Make A Big Difference.* Little, Brown, and Co., Hachette Book Group, New York, NY.

Mold JW. (2017) *Achieving Your Personal Health Goals: A Patient's Guide*. Full Court Press, Chapel Hill, NC.

Wagner EH. (1998) Chronic disease management: What will it take to improve care for chronic illness? *Portico Access, Effective Clinical Practice* 1: 2-4. **Chapter 1a**

Nussbaum AM. (2016) *The Finest Traditions of My Calling: One Physician's Search for the Renewal of Medicine*. Yale University Press, New Haven, CT.

Pollan M. (2006) *The Omnivore's Dilemma*. The Penguin Press, New York, NY.

Bortz WM. (1982) Disuse and Aging. *Journal of the American Medical Association*, 248(10): 1203-1208.

Crowley C and Lodge HS. (2005) *Younger Next Year: Live Strong, Fit, and Sexy – Until You're 80 and Beyond*. Workman Publishing, New York, NY.

National Academy of Medicine. (1999) *To Err is Human: Building a Safer Health System*. National Academy Press Washington, D.C.

CDC: Smoking and Tobacco Use, Tobacco-Related Mortality. *https://www.cdc.gov/tobacco/data_statistics/fact_sheets/health_effects/tobacco_related_mortality/index.htm*

Rehm J, Gmel G, Sempos CT, and Trevisan M. Alcohol-related morbidity and mortality. Chronic Consequences of Alcohol Use. National Institute on Alcohol Abuse and Addiction. *https://pubs. niaaa. nih.gov/publications/arh27-1/39-51.htm*

Welborn TL, Azarian MH, Davis N, Layton JC, Aspy C, and Mold JW. (2010) Development of an obesity counseling model based upon a study of determinants of intentional sustained weight loss. *Journal of the Oklahoma State Medical Association*, 103(7): 243-247.

Zirk-SadowskiJ, Masoli JA, Delgado J, et al. (2008) Proton pump inhibitors and long-term risk of community-acquired pneumonia in older adults. *Journal of the American Geriatrics Society*, 66(7): 1332-1338.

Nagykaldi Z, Aspy CB, Chou A, and Mold JW. (2012) Impact of a Wellness Portal on the delivery of patient-centered preventive care. *Journal of the American Board of Family Medicine*, 25(2): 158-166.

Nagykaldi ZJ, Voncken-Brewster V, Aspy CB, and Mold JW. (2013) Novel computerized health risk appraisal may improve longitudinal health and wellness in primary care. *Applied Clinical Informatics*, 5(4): 75-87.

Yarnall KSH, Pollak KI, Ostbye T, Krause KM, and Michener JL. (2003) Primary care: Is there enough time for prevention? *American Journal of Public Health*, 93(4): 635-641.

Ostbye T, Yarnall KSH, Krause KM, Pollak KI, Gradison M, and Michener JL. (2005) Is there time for management of patients with chronic diseases in primary care? *Annals of Family Medicine*, 3(3): 209-214.

SHEP Cooperative Research Group. (1991) Prevention of stroke by antihypertensive drug treatment in older persons with isolated systolic hypertension: final results of the Systolic Hypertension in the Elderly Program (SHEP). *Journal of the American Medical Association*, 265:3255-3264.

Shmagel A, Foley R, and Hassan I. (2016) Epidemiology of chronic low back pain in US adults: National Health and Nutrition Examination Survey 2009–2010. *Arthritis Care Research (Hoboken)*, 68(11): 1688–1694.

Chapter 1b

Mold JW, Hamm RM, and McCarthy LH. (2010) The law of diminishing returns in clinical medicine: How much risk reduction is enough? *Journal of the American Board of Family Medicine*, 23: 371-375.

Johnson HA. (1991) Diminishing returns on the road to diagnostic certainty. *Journal of the American Medical Association*, 65(17): 2229-2231.

Chapter 2a

McKenzie. (2011) *Treat Your Own Back* (9th ed.). Spinal Publications New Zealand.

Payer L. (1992) *Disease-Mongers: How Doctors, Drug Companies, and Insurers Are Making You Feel Sick.* John Wiley and Sons, Hoboken, NJ.

Moynihan R. and Cassels A. (2005) *Selling Sickness: How the World's Biggest Pharmaceutical Companies are Turning Us All into Patients.* Bold Type Books, Hachette Book Group, New York, NY.

Chapter 2b

No citations

Chapter 3

Erikson EH & Erikson JM. (1998) *The Life Cycle Completed.* Norton, New York, NY.

Pink DH. (2009) *Drive: The Surprising Truth About What Motivates Us.* Riverhead Books, New York, NY.

Chapter 4

Field M, and Cassell C. (1997) *Approaching death: improving care at the end of life* (IOM Report). National Academy Press, Washington, DC.

Emanuel EJ, and Emanuel LL. (1998) The promise of a good death. *Lancet*, 251: 21–29.

Mold JW, Looney S, Viviani NJ, and Quiggins PA. (1994) Predicting the health-related values and preferences of geriatric patients. *Journal of Family Practice*, 39:461-467.

Doukas DJ ,and McCulough LB. (1991) The Values History.The Evaluation of the Patient's Values and Advance Directives. *Journal of Family Practice* 32(2):145-53.

Gawande A. (2014) *Being Mortal: Medicine and What Matters in the*

End. Metropolitan Books, Henry Holt and Company, New York, NY.

Chapter 5

Berwick DM. (2020) To Isaiah. *Journal of the American Medical Association* 323(17): 1663-1665.

Chapter 6

Weed, LL. (1971) *Medical Records, Medical Education, and Patient Care: The Problem-Oriented Medical Record as a Basic Tool*. Cleveland, Ohio: Press of Case Western Reserve University.

Weed LL. (1991) *Knowledge Coupling: New Promises and New Tools for Medical Care and Education*. Springer-Verlag.

Chapter 7

No citations

Chapter 8

Wennberg J, and Gittelsohn A. (1973) Small area variations in health care delivery. *Science,* 182(4117): 1102-8.

Wennberg JE, and Cooper MM. (1996) *Dartmouth Atlas of Healthcare in the United States*. American Hospital Publishing Inc., Chicago, Il.

Boyd CM, Darer J, Boult C, Fried LP, Boult L, and Wu AW. (2005) Clinical Practice Guidelines and Quality of Care for Older Patients With Multiple Comorbid Diseases: Implications for Pay for Performance. *Journal of the American Medical Association,* 294(6): 716-724.

World Health Organization. (2016) *International Classification of Functioning, Disability and Health (ICF)*. Geneva, Switzerland.

Chapter 9

Pritt BS, Hardin NJ, Richmond JA, and Shapiro SI. (2005) Death certification errors at an academic institution. *Archives of Pathology and Laboratory Medicine,* 129(11): 1476-1479.

Cambridge B, and Cina SJ. (2010) The accuracy of death certificate completion in a suburban community. *American Journal of Forensic Medicine and Pathology*, 31(3): 232-235.

Wexelman BA, Eden E, and Rose KM. (2013) Survey of New York City resident physicians on case-of-death reporting, 2010. *Preventing Chronic Disease: Public Health Research, Practice, and Policy*, 10: E76. http://dx.doi.org/10.5888/pcd10.120288

McGivern L, Shulman L, Carney JK, Shapiro S, and Bundock E. (2017) Death certification errors and the effect on mortality statistics. *Public Health Reports*, 132(6): 669-675.

Alfsen GC, and Maelen J. (2012) The value of autopsies for determining the cause of death. *Journal of the Norwegian Medical Association*, 132: 147-151.

Winters B, Custer J, Galvagno Jr. SM, Colantuoni E, Kapoor SG, Lee H, et al. (2012) Diagnostic errors in the intensive care unit: A systematic review of autopsy studies. *British Medical Journal of Quality and Safety*, 21(11): 894-902.

Chapter 10

Purkaple BA, Mold JW, and Chen S. (2016) Encouraging patient-centered care by including quality-of-life questions on pre-encounter forms. *Annals of Family Medicine*, 14(3): 221-226.

Purkaple BA, Nagykaldi ZJ, Allahyar A, Todd R, Mold JW. (2020) Physicians' Response to Patients' Quality-of-Life Goals. *Journal of the American Board of Family Medicine*, 33: 71–79.

Chapter 11

World Health Organization. (1978) International Conference on Primary Care. Alma Ata Declaration. *WHO Chronicles*, 32(11): 428-430.

CDC Public Health Professionals Gateway: Community Health Assessment and Health Improvement Planning. *https://www.cdc.gov/pub-*

lichealthgateway/cha/index.html

Centers for Medicare and Medicaid Services. CMS Hospital Community Needs Assessment Process/Requirements. *https://www.cms.gov/ Outreach-and-Education/American-Indian-Alaska-Native/AIAN/ LTSS-TA-Center/planning/step-1-needs-assessment.*

Chapter 12

No citations

Chapter 13

No citations

Chapter 14a

Bortz WM Jr. (1984) The disuse syndrome. *Western Journal of Medicine*, 141(5):691-4.

Bortz WM Jr. (1993) The physics of frailty. *Journal of the American Geriatrics Society*, 41: 1004-1008.

Bortz W, IV and Bortz W, Jr. (1996) How fast do we age? Exercise performance over time as a biomarker. *Journal of Gerontology Medical Sciences*, 51: M223 -M225.

Bortz WM Jr. (2002) A conceptual framework of frailty: A review. *The Journals of Gerontology: Series A,* 57(5): M283–M288.

Chapter 14b

American Psychological Association: *https://www.apa.org/topics/resilience.*

Ryan RM, and Deci EL. (2000) Self Determination Theory and the facilitation of intrinsic motivation, social development, and well-being. *American Psychologist,* 55(1): 68-78.

Gladwell M. (2008) *Outliers: The Story of Success.* Little, Brown and Co., Hatchette Book Group, New York, NY.

Loudenback T. (2018) Spanx founder Sara Blakely learned an important lesson from her dad – Now she is passing it on to her 4 kids. *Business Insider*, Jun 17. *https://www.businessinsider.com/spanx-founder-sara-blakely-redefine-failure-2016-10*

Bethel CD, Gombojav N, and Whitaker RC. (2019) Family resilience and connection promote flourishing among U.S. children, even amid adversity. *Health Affairs*, 38(5): 729-737.

Gmuca S, Xiao R, Urquhart A, Weiss PF, Gillham JE, Ginsburg KR, Sherry DD, and Gerber JS. (2019) The role of patient and parental resilience in adolescents with chronic musculoskeletal pain. *Journal of Pediatrics*, 210: 118-126.

Liptak JJ, and Leubenberg ERA. (2012) *Teen Resiliency-Building Workbook*. Whole Person, Duluth, Minnesota, 2012.

Rosenberg AR, Bradford MC, Junkins CC, et al. (2019) Effect of promoting resilience in stress management intervention for parents of children with cancer (PRISM-P): A randomized clinical trial. *Journal of the American Medical Association Network Open*, 2(9): e1911578.

Lorig KR, Sobel D, Ritter PL, Hobbs M, Laurent D. (2001) Effect of a self-management program on patients with chronic disease. *Effective Clinical Practice*, 4: 256-262.

Lorig K, Sobel DS, Stewart AL, Brown BW, Bandura A, Ritter P, González VM, Laurent DD, and Holman HR. (1999) Evidence suggesting that a chronic disease self-management program can improve health status while reducing hospitalization: a randomized trial. *Medical Care*, 37(1): 5-14.

Coleman EA, Smith JD, Frank JC, Min SJ, Parry C, and Kramer AM. (2004) Preparing patients and caregivers to participate in care delivered across settings: the Care Transitions Intervention. *Journal of the American Geriatrics Society,* 52(11):1817-1825.

Boehmer KR, Guerton NM, Soyring J, Hargraves I, Dick S, and Montori V. (2019) Capacity Coaching: A New Strategy for Coaching Patients Living With Multimorbidity and Organizing Their Care. *Mayo Clinic Proceedings*, 94(2): 278-286.

Valdivia J. A Buddhist approach to resilience. *https://medium.com/@jeff.valdivia/a-buddhist-approach-to-resilience-a73280ff39fc*

Chapter 15

Iannuzzi MC, Rybicki BA, and Tierstein AS. Sarcoidosis. (2007) *New England Journal of Medicine*, 357: 2153-2165.

Rogers, C. (1951) *Client-centered Therapy: Its Current Practice, Implications and Theory*. Constable, London.

Stewart M. (1995) *Patient-Centered Medicine: Transforming the Clinical Method*. Radcliffe Medical Press Ltd, Abingdon, UK.

Charon R. (2006) *Narrative Medicine: Honoring the Stories of Illness*. Oxford University Press, New York, NY.

Chapter 16

Eddy D and Cohen M. (2011) Description of the Archimedes Model: ARCHeS Simulator 2.3. *Archimedes Quantifying Healthcare*, 1-57. *https://journals.plos.org/plosone/article/file?type=supplementary&id=info:doi/10.1371/journal.pone.0066454.s002*